Skills and Techniques for Human Service Professionals

Counseling Environment, Helping Skills,

Treatment Issues

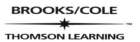

ED NEUKRUG
Old Dominion University

BROOKS/COLE

TM

THOMSON LEARNING

Australia • Canada • Mexico • Singapore • Spain • United Kingdom • United States

75.00

To My Wife, Kristina

BROOKS/COLE
✶
THOMSON LEARNING

Executive Acquisitions Editor: *Lisa Gebo*
Assistant Editor: *Alma Dea Michelena*
Marketing Team: *Carolyn Concilla, Megan Hansen, Tami Strang*
Editorial Assistant: *Sheila Walsh*
Project Editor: *Laurel Jackson*
Production Service: *Shepherd, Inc.*
Manuscript Editor: *Patterson Lamb*

Permissions Editor: *Sue Ewing*
Cover Design: *Christine Garrigan*
Cover Photos: *Corbis Images*
Interior Illustration: *Anne-Marie Gephart*
Print Buyer: *Nancy Panziera*
Typesetting: *Shepherd, Inc.*
Printing and Binding: *Webcom*

For more information about this or any other Brooks/Cole product, contact:
BROOKS/COLE
511 Forest Lodge Road
Pacific Grove, CA 93950 USA
www.brookscole.com
1-800-423-0563 (Thomson Learning Academic Resource Center)

For permission to use material from this work, contact us by
www.thomsonrights.com
fax: 1-800-730-2215
phone: 1-800-730-2214

Printed in Canada

10 9 8 7 6 5

Library of Congress Cataloging-in-Publication Data

Neukrug, Ed.
    Skills and techniques for human service professionals : counseling environment, helping skills, treatment issues / Ed Neukrug.—1st ed.
        p. cm.
    Includes bibliographical references and index.
    ISBN-13: 978-0-534-56768-2
    ISBN-10: 0-534-56768-1
    1. Human services. 2. Human services personnel. 3. Helping behavior. 4. Counseling.
    5. Counselor and client. I. Title.
HV40 .N44 2001
361'.06—dc21

2001035725

Contents

WITHDRAWN

Preface

Increasingly, as I have examined the kinds of helping skills texts that are used by human service professionals, I have found that they do not address the special roles and functions of this group. Often, these texts are written for programs outside the human services or focus on skills more appropriate for in-depth counseling and psychotherapy rather than on the kinds of helping skills practiced by human service professionals. Because I have held a number of positions in the helping professions and have written texts on both human services and counseling, I thought I might be able to create a text that addresses the unique roles and functions of the human service professional.

The goal of this book is to help students gain a thorough understanding of the attitudes, techniques and skills, and major treatment issues that are unique to the helping relationship in which the human service professional practices. This is reflected in the major divisions of the book. However, the approach is different in several ways. For one, an entire section is devoted to the impact of the helping environment—on both the application of the helper's skills and the client's experience of the helping relationship. This element is often overlooked but is extremely important.

Another difference is the practical approach to discussing and teaching specific skills. They are presented in a down-to-earth manner and are accompanied by many exercises, making this truly a hands-on book. In addition, there are vignettes that can be used to stimulate discussion, as well as ethical and professional dilemmas that invite student reflection. Also, at the end of each chapter are questions that can be researched through InfoTrac® College Edition.

The text works best if the class becomes really involved in the activities and the instructor takes an active learning approach with the students. By moving away from a didactic, pedagogical style, the activities should create an enjoyable learning environment for both students and faculty. When you finish the book, I hope you agree with my six-year-old daughter, Hannah, who says that "learning is fun, and I hope you think it's fun, too!"

To help the instructor adapt the text to each class, an instructor's manual with chapter outlines, overheads, and test bank is available online at: http://www.wadsworth.com/humansvcs_d/.

Acknowledgments

I would like to thank the following reviewers for their insightful comments and suggestions: Susan Kerstein, National-Louis University, Evanston Campus; Rob Lawson, Western Washington University; Alvin Lewis, Pima Community College; Barbara Peterson, Tacoma Community College; and Cynthia Poindexter, Boston University.

I'd like to give a special thanks to my wife, Kristina, for her tireless efforts editing the manuscript. Also, I would like to thank Debra Boyce for assisting with the Table of Contents and Index, and for helping me with dozens of inane editing questions. A special thanks also goes to the following individuals: Peggy Francomb from Shepherd, Inc. for coordinating the many aspects of this book, and for being there when I needed some assistance; Alma Dea Michelena from Brooks/Cole for giving me some excellent suggestions in restructuring the text; and Lisa Gebo from Brooks/Cole for her continued support, encouragement, and friendship.

Ed Neukrug

Introduction

The work of the human service professional is generally focused around one or more of 13 roles and functions identified by the Southern Regional Education Board (SREB, 1969). These include the following:

1. *Outreach* worker who might go into communities to work with clients.
2. *Broker* who helps clients find and use services.
3. *Advocate* who champions and defends clients' causes and rights.
4. *Evaluator* who assesses client programs and shows that agencies are accountable for services provided.
5. *Teacher/educator* who tutors, mentors, and models new behaviors for clients.
6. *Behavior changer* who uses intervention strategies and counseling skills to facilitate client change.
7. *Mobilizer* who organizes client and community support in order to provide needed services.
8. *Consultant* who seeks and offers knowledge and support to other professionals and meets with clients and community groups to discuss and solve problems.
9. *Community planner* who designs, implements, and organizes new programs to service client needs.
10. *Caregiver* who offers direct support, encouragement, and hope to clients.
11. *Data manager* who develops systems to gather facts and statistics as a means of evaluating programs.
12. *Administrator* who supervises community service programs.
13. *Assistant to specialist* who works closely with the highly trained professional as an aide and helper in servicing clients (Schram & Mandel, 1997).

More recently, in a national project to develop skills standards, 12 competencies were identified as important to the work of the human service professional (Taylor, Bradly, & Warren, 1996). These include (1) participant empowerment; (2) communication; (3) assessment; (4) community and service networking; (5) facilitation of services; (6) community and living skills and supports; (7) education, training, and self-development; (8) advocacy; (9) vocational, educational, and career support; (10) crisis intervention; (11) organization participation; and (12) documentation.

The competencies are developed through acquisition of a set of skills or job functions reflected in activity statements or tasks that the human service practitioner would undertake to fulfill the job functions (Taylor, Bradly, & Warren, 1996).

COMPETENCY AREAS   →   SKILLS   →   TASKS
                              (Job Functions)   (Activity Statements)

As one example, for the competency of "Communication," one skill would be to use "effective, sensitive, communication skills to build rapport" (Taylor, Bradly, & Warren, 1996, p. 26), and one activity instrumental to accomplishing this skill is the use of active listening skills. Appendix A defines the 12 competency areas.

The purpose of this book is to identify many of the skills and techniques necessary for successful implementation of the roles, functions, and competencies of the human service professional as identified by SREB and by the skills standards project. In that effort, the text is divided into three sections: Section I is focused on the counseling environment, Section II on helping skills, and Section III on treatment issues.

SECTION I: THE COUNSELING ENVIRONMENT

Chapter 1, "Characteristics of the Effective Helper," briefly examines characteristics that human service professionals should avoid and then focuses on eight personality characteristics that seem to be related to positive client outcomes. These include being empathic, being open, being real, having high internality, being an experiencer of life, having good emotional health, being an alliance builder, and having competence. The importance of embracing these characteristics is discussed, as is the notion that human service professionals must strive continually to embody these characteristics as they progress in their careers.

Chapter 2, "Entering the Agency," considers how the client experiences the agency during the initial contact, how the client is affected by the atmosphere of the helper's office, and how nonverbal behaviors affect the client. Such nonverbal behaviors include the helper's attire, eye contact, body positioning and facial expressions, personal space, touch, and voice intonation and tone. The chapter concludes with a discussion of the importance to helpers of being aware of cross-cultural differences in nonverbal behavior.

SECTION II: HELPING SKILLS

Chapter 3, "Stages of the Helping Relationship: Theories, Process, and Skills," opens the second section by offering a model for understanding the relationships among theory, case conceptualization, stages of the helping relationship, and the skills used within the helping relationship. After a brief overview of five theoretical orientations—psychodynamic, humanistic, behavioral, cognitive, and brief treatment—the relationship between theory and one's view of human nature is explored. This is followed by an examination of the stages of the helping relationship and the various helping skills that may be appropriate for use within each one. The stages include the pre-interview stage, the rapport and trust-building stage, the problem-identification stage, the goal-setting stage, the work stage, the closure stage, and the post-relationship stage: the revolving door. Throughout the chapter, the complex relationship among theory, stage, and skills is highlighted.

Chapter 4, "Foundational Skills," deals with skills that are fundamental to the helping relationship. These are crucial in establishing the relationship, building rapport and trust, setting a tone with the client, and beginning the client's process of self-examination. They include using silence effectively, having good listening skills, and showing appropriate empathy to clients.

Chapter 5, "Commonly Used Skills," focuses on skills frequently used by many helpers to build a strong foundation for the helping relationship. Compared to listening and empathy, in which the client is free to choose what he or she wishes to discuss, the skills in this chapter guide the client toward certain topics. Thus, the skills of affirmation and encouragement direct clients by reinforcing what they are discussing, and the skills of modeling and self-disclosure encourage clients to focus on specific topics that the helper is modeling or revealing about himself or herself.

Section II continues with the skills involved in collecting information from clients. Chapter 6, "Information Gathering," distinguishes among direct, closed, open, and tentative questions. The use of "why" questions is explored, and when to use questions, as well as the pros and cons of their use, is presented. The second part of this chapter is concerned with gathering information using a structured interview. Increasingly, a large amount of information is elicited from clients when they first enter an agency, and the structured interview is an efficient method for gathering this information in a timely and thorough fashion.

Chapter 7, "Helper-Centered Skills," examines a number of different skills that helpers use in leading the session. First, the solution-centered skills of offering alternatives, giving advice, and providing information are demonstrated. Next, offering feedback to clients through confrontation and interpretation is explored. Finally, the use of token economies and other specialized skills is briefly touched on.

SECTION III: TREATMENT ISSUES

Chapter 8, "Case Management," presents nine major aspects of managing a caseload. The first is treatment planning, which includes how to assess clients' needs and the relationship between assessing needs and developing goals. Next, the process of diagnosing clients, with particular emphasis on the *Diagnostic and Statistical Manual of Mental Disorders* (DSM-IV-TR) (American Psychiatric Association, 2000), is examined. The use of psychotropic drugs, with particular focus on antipsychotic, antimanic, antidepressant, and antianxiety agents and stimulants is the next area of case management that is explored. Case report writing, the fourth aspect, discusses writing case reports and mental status reports and examines the ethical and legal issues related to case report writing. The last five aspects of case management examined are managing and documenting client contact hours; monitoring, evaluating, and documenting progress toward client goals; making referrals; handling follow-up; and using time management.

Chapter 9, "Multicultural Counseling: Issues and Techniques," focuses on cross-cultural counseling, an increasingly important aspect of the human service profession. This chapter states why multicultural issues are so crucial at this time and explains why counseling often does not work for many members of minority groups. Next, an existential model of understanding the culturally diverse client is presented. The model emphasizes the point that, to be effective in cross-cultural relationships, helpers must possess appropriate beliefs, attitudes, knowledge, and skills. The second part of the chapter stresses specific points to consider when working with a wide range of clients, including individuals from different ethnic and racial groups, diverse religious backgrounds, gay men and lesbians, individuals who are HIV positive, the homeless and the poor, older persons, people with mental illness, and individuals with disabilities.

The last chapter of this book, "Ethical and Professional Issues," reviews important ethical, professional, and legal issues in the human service profession. First, the purpose of ethical guidelines and the ethical decision-making process are discussed. A good part of the chapter then focuses on some of the more important ethical and professional issues that human service professionals face. Each issue is followed by ethical vignettes appropriate to the issue that was discussed. Specific ethical issues to be studied include informed consent, competence and scope of knowledge, supervision, confidentiality, privileged communication, dual relationships, sexual relationships with clients, primary obligation, continuing education, and multicultural issues.

Skills and Techniques for Human Service Professionals is designed to help students gain a comprehensive understanding of important skills unique to the human service professional. Within the text, you will find new approaches to the application of traditional skills, vignettes that highlight the learning experience, and hands-on activities that will help you practice and learn important skills and concepts. I hope you learn from the text and enjoy the activities in it.

Ed Neukrug

SECTION I

The Counseling Environment

A successful helping relationship needs a nurturing environment, one in which clients feel comfortable and welcome. Many elements in an environment can affect a client positively or negatively, and some of these are seldom given conscious attention. One is the personal characteristics, behavior, and dress of the particular helper the client will work with. In so many aspects of who he or she is, a helper can project a casual, not particularly caring attitude, or warmth, empathy, and understanding. Another is the first impression the client receives as he or she enters the agency; this initial experience is very important to clients as they sense what to expect and how they will be treated in the agency. The elements that make up the environment of the helping relationship and their effect on it—for good or ill—are discussed in the chapters of this section.

1

Characteristics
of the Effective Helper

INTRODUCTION

Did you ever listen to Dr. Laura, the radio talk show host? She is critical, dogmatic, and moralistic. Nevertheless, she is one of the most popular radio talk show hosts on the air! There is something about her personality style that draws people to listen to her. However, being a "draw" doesn't mean she embodies the characteristics of the human service professional that are typically considered to be important. To be effective, this professional needs to know what skills work as well as have the personality to use these skills successfully.

In this chapter, I discuss qualities that human service professionals should avoid, then introduce eight personality traits that have shown to be related to positive client outcomes. As you read through the chapter, consider the characteristics Dr. Laura seems to embrace and reflect on your own personality. If you find that most of the characteristics in this chapter *do not* describe you, then you, like most people, will probably have to work hard to incorporate these qualities into your personality. However, if you believe these qualities are important, then over time they will become a natural part of you, and your journey to becoming an effective helper will begin.

HELPER QUALITIES TO AVOID AND TO EMBRACE

The effective helper must avoid attitudes and behaviors that will foster a destructive relationship. For example, the helper who continually makes empathic failures is not hearing the client. The helper who seems false, judgmental, and dogmatic creates defensiveness in the client. The helper who is externally oriented does not appear grounded in the session. The impaired helper's unfinished business interferes with client growth. The helper who cannot build an alliance leaves the client floundering, and the helper who lacks appropriate knowledge and skills can hardly be competent.

There are many other behaviors and attitudes that a helper could display that would be detrimental to a helping relationship: being critical, disapproving, or disbelieving; scolding, threatening, discounting, ridiculing, or punishing; being sexist; showing prejudice; and being rejecting toward a client (Benjamin, 1987). All of these need to be avoided in the helping relationship, but there are many qualities that the helper should actively exhibit. Let's now take a look at some of these.

Over the years, research has shown a number of traits to be important in building a successful helping relationship (Gladstein, 1983; Highlen & Hill, 1984; Lambert, Shapiro, & Bergin, 1986; Neukrug & McAuliffe, 1993; Rowe, Murphy, De Csipkes, 1975; Sexton, 1993; Sexton & Whiston, 1991, 1994). The eight characteristics that seem to be either empirically or theoretically related to effectiveness as a helper include (1) being empathic, (2) being open, (3) being real, (4) having high internality, (5) being an experiencer of life, (6) having good emotional health, (7) being an alliance builder, (8) being competent.

THE EIGHT CHARACTERISTICS

Being Empathic

Empathic individuals have a deep understanding of another person's point of view. These people can "get inside another person's shoes." For those of you who have watched *Star Trek: The Next Generation,* the "counselor" character is the epitome of the empathic person with her ability to merge with the experience of the person she is attempting to understand. Carl Rogers (1957), probably the best-known humanistic psychologist, liked to state that the empathic person could sense the private world of the client as if it were his or her own, without losing the "as if" feeling. Empathic individuals accept people's differences and communicate this sense of acceptance. In respect to the helping relationship, empathy is a skill that can build rapport, elicit information, and help the client feel accepted (Carkhuff, 2000; Egan, 2001). Being empathic can be operationalized; that is, it can be described in a manner that can be measured. In Chapter 4, empathy is examined as a skill and ways to apply this skill in the helping relationship are discussed. To see how empathic you are at present, do Exercise 1.1.

EXERCISE 1.1   Are You Empathic?

Separate into triads and label one person "Number 1," the second person "Number 2," and the last person, "Number 3." Number 1 begins by talking with Number 2 about an emotionally charged situation he or she has experienced in his or her life. Number 1 should attempt to be as real as possible in relating the situation while Number 2 should respond by trying to be as empathic as possible. Number 3 will record the session on audio- or videotape. After about 10 minutes, listen to the tape and discuss the situation using the checklist below. After Number 1 and Number 2 have finished, Number 2 should be paired up with Number 3, with Number 2 describing a situation and Number 3 trying to be empathic (Number 1 records). Finally, when they have finished, Number 3 and Number 1 are paired up, with Number 3 describing a situation, Number 1 being empathic, and Number 2 recording the session.

After completing the exercise, all three individuals in the group will listen to each tape together. Using the rating scale below, they will discuss each item within the small group and decide, for each tape, one group rating score for each item. After they have completed the ratings, they will average the six items.

1	2	3	4	5
not at all like this (not empathic)		somewhere in the middle		very much like this (empathic)

1. *Talks minimally:* The empathic person will talk considerably less than the individual who is describing the situation.
2. *Asks few questions:* The empathic person will tend to ask few, if any questions.
3. *Does not offer advice:* The empathic person will give little if any advice.
4. *Does not judge:* The empathic person will not judge the person he or she is listening to.
5. *Does not interpret:* The empathic person will not analyze and/or interpret the other person's situation.
6. *Does not cut off:* The empathic person will not cut off the other person and will allow himself or herself to be cut off by the person talking.

If after scoring the responses, the group has an average that is more than 3.0 (the ratings were mostly 3s, 4s, and 5s), they are doing very well. If, however, their average is lower than 3 (the ratings were mostly 1s, 2s, or 3s), they have work to do. Chapter 4 examines the skill of empathy in more depth and offers the opportunity to fine-tune this important response.

Being Open

Individuals who are open to others are accepting and able to allow others to express their points of view. These individuals do not feel as if they need to change others to their way of viewing the world. Such nondogmatic individuals are open to criticism, open to change, and open to hearing and understanding the views of others in a way that will allow them to reflect on their own values and beliefs. Individuals who are open to others are relatively free from biases and can accept people's differences, regardless of dissimilar cultural heritage, values, or belief systems.

Although most of us have strong convictions about certain issues, generally we don't go around trying to convince people to change to our point of view. If we do spend a lot of energy trying to change others, it is probably because we have closed ourselves off from hearing other views. Such lack of openness can prevent us from listening effectively to another person. If I am spending all my energy trying to convince someone to embrace my beliefs, how can I hear that person? In fact, some research shows a relationship between being nondogmatic, or open to others, and being a good listener (Neukrug & McAuliffe, 1993).

In a helping relationship, individuals who are open to another's experience are able to accept the helpee (the person needing help) unconditionally, without having "strings attached" to the relationship. Rogers (1957) calls this unconditional positive regard. Leo Buscaglia calls this responsible love:

> Responsible love is accepting and understanding. . . . [L]ove helps us to accept the fact that the other individual is behaving only as he [or she] is able to behave at the moment" (1972, p. 119).

Exercise 1.2 can help you see how open you are.

Being Real

People can generally tell when a person is "real" or when someone is "throwing them a line." Real people are "together" in the sense that they are aware of their feelings and are willing to express them through their thoughts and actions, when appropriate. On the other hand, nongenuine people are not in touch with their feelings and how they feel is not represented by what they say or how they act. These individuals are fake, living life with subtle deceptions, often deceiving themselves. Unless people are thoroughly caught up in a nongenuine way of living, they usually have a sense that they are behaving incongruently—that is, that their feelings, thoughts, and behaviors are not consistent. There is a slight (sometimes more than slight) internal tug saying "something's not right inside" or "I know I'm trying to put something over on this person."

Rogers (1961, 1980) believed that genuineness was a crucial element in both the helping relationship and in *all* of life's relationships. He thus expressed the opinion that helpers must model realness. Rogers and others assert that those who are genuine are transparent; that is, they readily show their feelings to others (Greenberg, 1994; Jourard, 1971; Rogers, 1957). Recognizing the importance of this quality, Gelso and Carter (1994) believe that every helping relationship must address this important issue. For instance, they believe that those helpers who do not reveal themselves during a helping relationship must somehow deal with how their clients will react to the wall they put up.

Peck (1998) discussed the importance of being real for the client. He stated that "small white lies" could snowball over time, become a nongenuine lifestyle, and eventually represent evil. He even felt that this nongenuine lifestyle could take over one's life. Most people would agree that living a nongenuine lifestyle is not healthy. Peck believed that a helper who is genuine can facilitate realness in the client. He saw the helping relationship as holding the same power

---

EXERCISE 1.2   How Open Are You?

In class, divide into triads. From the list below, find a situation in which one person is "pro" and one person is "con." If for the situations listed all of your group is either "pro" or "con," try to come up with a situation in which one of you is pro and one is con. Your task is to have one person who is pro and one who is con discuss the situation. The third person is the "moderator" who should take notes and later give feedback as to how each individual is responding to the role-play. While discussing the situation, try your best to listen to the other person's point of view. When you have finished, discuss the points listed below. Then, repeat the situation, or do another situation, but this time the moderator is pro or con and one of the other individuals is the moderator. When you have finished, answer the questions listed that follow.

Situations

1. Abortion
2. Increased taxes
3. Affirmative action
4. Opening an X-rated bookstore in your neighborhood
5. Capital punishment
6. National health insurance
7. Increased tuition

Points to Consider

1. Did you become so emotionally charged about the situation that you were unable to hear the other person (closed to the person)?
2. Did you think the other person was "wrong."
3. Did you get tense while discussing the situation?
4. Did the individual with whom you were discussing the situation consider you open or closed to his or her point of view?
5. Did the "moderator" consider you to be open or closed?
6. Did you think you were open or closed?
7. Did you tend to cut off the other person from talking?
8. Were you preoccupied with trying to come up with a response in order to refute what the other person was saying?
9. Did the other person's point of view make sense to you?
10. Did you consider changing your point of view based on what you heard?

If you answered "yes" to many of items 1 through 8, and "no" to items 9 and 10, then you were probably somewhat closed and nonaccepting. Although you might act differently in the role of helper, this exercise gives you some sense of how open you are.

---

as a "mini-confessional," in which people can cleanse themselves of their incongruities. Exercise 1.3 can help you look at one aspect of being real.

Having High Internality

Before you go any further, complete Exercise 1.4.

If in Exercise 1.4 your line falls in Quandrant I, then you have a high degree of internality, which can be viewed as a combination of a high locus of control and a high degree of responsibility taking. Individuals who have a high

---

EXERCISE 1.3   Keeping Secrets

Keeping secrets is one way that we prevent ourselves from being real with another person. In the space provided, make a list of secrets you have kept from significant people in your life. Then answer the questions given. When you have finished, without necessarily talking specifically about any one secret, in small groups, discuss what you discovered about your secrets.

1._____

2._____

3._____

4._____

5._____

6._____

7._____

8._____

9._____

10._____

Questions
1. Was it relatively easy to remember 10 secrets?
2. Why have you kept these secrets?
3. Have you found it easier to keep these secrets than confront the person from whom you are holding the secret?
4. What benefits do you derive from keeping each secret?
5. What are the drawbacks to keeping each secret?
6. What is your best course of action for each secret?
7. What might happen if the secret(s) was (were) revealed?

---

degree of internality place more importance on internal thoughts and beliefs and are not significantly persuaded by others—although they may take other people's opinions into account in decision making. Research shows that people who have a high degree of internality do not have a need to convince others of how to be (Neukrug & McAuliffe, 1993). However, too much internality can be unhealthy, and Shostrum (1974) notes that healthy individuals have a 3:1 ratio of "inner directedness to other directedness." This means they mostly rely on themselves in decision making, take pride in listening to themselves and taking responsibility for themselves, but are also willing to consider the viewpoints of others.

In the professional world, much importance is placed on internality, and a human service professional will likely do well if he or she has a high degree of internality. And, most clients will do well with a higher degree of responsibility and locus of control. However, keep in mind that internality is a particularly

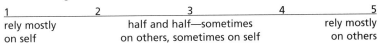

EXERCISE 1.4   Locus of Control and Locus of Responsibility

1. Rate yourself on how responsible you view yourself.

1	2	3	4	5
extremely responsible		moderately responsible		not at all responsible

2. Rate yourself on whether you tend to rely more on yourself or on others when making decisions.

1	2	3	4	5
rely mostly on self		half and half—sometimes on others, sometimes on self		rely mostly on others

Now, taking the scores you gave yourself, circle the appropriate number in the figure that follows. Your score on question 1 should be placed on the *X* (horizontal) axis and your score on question 2 on the *Y* (vertical) axis. Then draw a line that connects the two numbers.

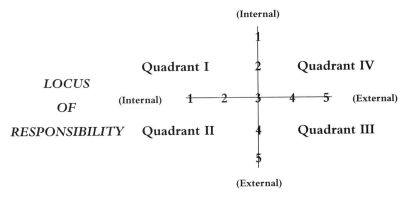

LOCUS OF CONTROL

(Internal)

Quadrant I   Quadrant IV

LOCUS

OF   (Internal)   1   2   3   4   5   (External)

RESPONSIBILITY   Quadrant II   Quadrant III

(External)

SOURCE: Adapted from "Counseling Across Cultures," by D. W. Sue, 1978, *Personnel and Guidance Journal, 56,* 460. Copyright © 1978 American Counseling Association. Reprinted with permission. No further reproduction authorized without written permission.

Western value and may not be embraced by some clients from non-Western backgrounds (Pedersen, 2000; Sue, 1978; Yutrzenka, 1995). For instance, an individual who has a family that deeply values listening to the advice of elders may fall into one of the other quadrants.

Falling in a different quadrant becomes pathological only when rigid adherence to a style results in negative consequences, such as a high degree of anxiety or depression. Indeed, although Americans tend to favor the style of relating reflected by Quadrant I, falling into a different quadrant is not necessarily bad. As Americans, we tend to value Quadrant I behavior, and many clients will thrive with increased internality, but we also must not confuse such behavior as ultimately the *right* way to be.

EXERCISE 1.5   Allowing Yourself to Experience

Pair up with another person in your class. Have one person reflect on a problem situation in his or her life and then give the situation a title. For instance, if I was concerned about my work relationship with a colleague, I might call it "Problems with Jerrad." Next, in one minute tell your situation to the person with whom you're paired. The instructor should time you. Then do the same exercise, but this time give yourselves 5 to 10 minutes to discuss the situation. If time allows, have the other person in the dyad do the same task with his or her own unique situation. After you have finished, make notes about the following:

1. What differences did you find in your understanding of the problem after 10 minutes as compared to 5 minutes?
2. Did you find that there were "layers" to the problem? For instance, problems with Jerrad might be more related to problems I have relating to male colleagues, which might be related to problems I had relating to my dad.
3. Did you find that you experienced deeper, more profound feelings when you had more time to discuss the problem?

After students have reflected on these three questions, the instructor should ask the class to discuss what they found. Individuals could volunteer to discuss their responses to the items above.

Being an Experiencer of Life

Do Exercise 1.5.

Rush, rush, rush. This is a high-stress, high-rush world we live in. As the cliché goes, so often we don't even take time to smell the roses. Slow down, take time to experience life—enjoy what you have, make goals for what you want, live.

> I remembered one morning when I discovered a cocoon in the bark of a tree, just as a butterfly was making a hole in its case and preparing to come out. I waited a while, but it was too long appearing and I was impatient. I bent over it and breathed on it to warm it. I warmed it as quickly as I could and the miracle began to happen before my eyes, faster than life. The case opened, the butterfly started slowly crawling out and I shall never forget my horror when I saw how its wings were folded back and crumpled; the wretched butterfly tried with its whole trembling body to unfold them. Bending over it, I tried to help it with my breath. In vain. It needed to be hatched out patiently and the unfolding of the wings should be a gradual process in the sun. Now it was too late. My breath had forced the butterfly to appear, all crumpled, before its time. It struggled desperately and, a few seconds later, died in the palm of my hand. That little body is, I do believe, the greatest weight I have on my conscience. For I realize today that it is a mortal sin to violate the great laws of nature. We should not hurry, we should not be impatient, but we should confidently obey the eternal rhythm. (Kazantzakis, 1952, pp. 120–121)

People who allow themselves to experience life are able to let life unfold naturally and can accept their feelings and thoughts in the moment. Helpers such as these view life as a blossoming process. They understand the importance of slowly allowing their client relationships to unfold; otherwise, much like the butterfly, their helping relationships will falter. Working with clients can be tedious, and change often occurs very slowly. It is important to be able to be in the moment with one's clients and to not push them too fast. Push a client too quickly, and you're likely to push him or her out of the helping relationship.

Having Good Emotional Health

Can you help others if you yourself need help? This is a crucial question that all helpers must ask themselves. Helpers, like all people, struggle with life's concerns, and a helper does not necessarily have to be on the top of the world to be effective. However, a seriously impaired helper is likely to have difficulty being effective with clients, and some studies have shown the emotional health of the helper is likely related to positive client outcomes (Lambert & Bergin, 1983). In addition, some research shows that positive client outcomes may be more likely if a helper has experienced his or her own personal counseling (Greenberg & Staller, 1981). With 66% to 84% of varying types of helping professionals having participated in their own counseling (Deutsch, 1984; Neukrug, Milliken, & Shoemaker, 2001; Neukrug & Williams, 1993; Norcross, Strausser, & Faltus, 1988; Pope & Tabachnick, 1994; Prochaska & Norcross, 1983), it is heartening to see that helpers seem to want to work on their own issues.

Participation in one's own counseling has a number of benefits for the budding helper. First, it obviously can assist the helper in dealing with his or her own personal difficulties. "For a counselor to set themselves up as a helper to others, without having resolved major difficulties of their own, would appear to be farcical" (Wheeler, 1991, p. 199). Second, the helper can experience firsthand those techniques that might seem most beneficial. Third, having been in counseling enables the helper to identify and empathize with what it's like to sit in the client's seat. Fourth, personal counseling yields great insight into self, which surely must have a positive effect on the helping relationship. Finally, a personal experience with counseling helps to prevent countertransference—the situation in which professionals overly identify with a client, project themselves onto the client, and meet their own needs through their clients (Corey, 2001). In fact, Gelso and Carter (1994) suggest that countertransference will play an important role in the health and development of the helping relationship, regardless of whether the helper is actively attending to it.

Is counseling the only road to emotional health? Probably not. However, it is a very special relationship that is not achievable through friendships or other significant relationships. Other activities such as support groups, meditation, exercise, and journaling have all been shown to have positive effects on one's emotional health, but personal counseling for helpers is one of a few activities that can lead to emotional health, more effective helping relationships, and strong therapeutic alliances with clients. Exercise 1.6 can help you see whether you are devoting sufficient time to your emotional health.

EXERCISE 1.6   Ways of Attaining and Maintaining Emotional Health

Make a list of the ways that you take care of yourself in an effort to maintain your emotional health. Share your list in a small group or with the class.

1. _____
2. _____
3. _____
4. _____
5. _____
6. _____
7. _____
8. _____
9. _____
10. _____

Being an Alliance Builder

Will you be able to connect with a client? If not, research seems to indicate that you may not be as effective a helper as someone who can (Sexton & Whiston, 1991, Whiston & Coker, 2000). But what does it mean to connect with a client? Do the following simple exercise (Exercise 1.7).

Building an alliance with a client is closely related to the ability of the client and helper to develop an emotional bond and to work on setting and attaining goals (Bordin, 1979). Whether or not it is acknowledged by the helper and/or client, the working alliance exists throughout the helping relationship (Gelso & Carter, 1994). The well-known family therapist Salvadore Minuchin (1974) stands apart from many other helpers in his acknowledgment and description of the importance of the alliance. Using the term *joining,* he notes that the helper must position himself or herself in a manner that will be conducive to connecting with clients so that ultimately the helper can influence the change process. The challenge for all helpers is to have the emotional fortitude to build strong alliances with their clients, to know how to build such bonds within the context of their theoretical framework, and to be able to understand how these bonds dramatically affect their work with clients.

Being Competent

Truly effective human service professionals have a thirst for knowledge and understand that knowledge is closely related to competence. They exhibit their quest for knowledge through their studies, their desire to join professional associations and read professional journals, and their ability to broaden and deepen their own approach with clients. Effective human service professionals under-

---

EXERCISE 1.7   Building Alliances with Others

Identify three to five people whom you trust to be honest in answering some questions about you. (You might want to use some of the people in your class who have worked with you on prior exercises, but you could also ask family and friends.) Tell the individuals you have chosen that you will be asking three to five people to respond to the same items, and that you will attempt to keep each person's answers anonymous (e.g., do not place names on each person's responses and wait until you have all responses before viewing them). Ask each person to answer the following items.

1. Most of the time, the person I am rating is
    (1) approachable
    (2) somewhat approachable
    (3) a little approachable
    (4) not too approachable
    (5) not at all approachable

2. When I talk with the person I am rating, he or she seems to be

1	2	3	4	5
interested in me		moderately interested in me		not at all interested in me

3. I can tell that the person I am rating generally wants to

1	2	3	4	5
connect with me		sometimes connect with me but sometimes not connect with me		not connect with me

4. The following are ways in which the person I am assessing shows me that he or she attempts to connect with me:

    (1) _____

    (2) _____

    (3) _____

    (4) _____

Take an average of the ratings for the first three questions, and then make a list of all of the items in question 4. For the first three items, it is likely that the closer you are to 1, the easier it is for you to build an alliance. Then examine the responses to item 4. Particularly look to see if any items in question 4 were identified by more than one person. This may indicate a primary way that you "connect" with others. Your instructor may ask you to discuss your results with others in the class or in small groups.

---

stand that some techniques are more effective than others with certain client populations, and such professionals have a desire to learn what works best with whom (Kanfer & Goldstein, 1991; Whiston & Coker, 2000).

Competent professionals view education as a lifelong process, and they believe that human service professionals have both an ethical and a legal responsibility to be competent (Corey, Corey, & Callanan, 1998). The *Ethical Standards of Human Service Professionals* (1995, see Appendix B) supports the importance for human service professionals of continuing to gain knowledge

---

EXERCISE 1.8   Competence

Place the appropriate number next to the item that seems most like you.
1. I very much *do not* agree with this statement
2. I *do not* agree with this statement
3. I neither agree nor disagree with this statement
4. I agree with this statement
5. I very much agree with this statement

___ 1. I love the learning that takes place in school.
___ 2. I often pick up books, journal articles, or other written materials concerning subjects I want to learn more about.
___ 3. I wish I didn't have to take classes and someone could just give me a college degree!
___ 4. I view learning as a lifelong process.
___ 5. I tend to be cynical in class.
___ 6. I have joined a professional association.
___ 7. When I have a job in my profession, I plan on becoming a member of a professional association.
___ 8. Research can add little about my knowledge of clients.
___ 9. When I write research papers, I do an exhaustive search of the literature.
___10. I believe that consulting with other professionals is generally a waste of time.

Scoring the inventory: For items 1, 2, 4, 6, 7, and 9, give yourself the number of points that you wrote in for that item. For items 3, 5, 8, and 10, if you answered "1" give yourself 5 points, "2" give yourself 4 points, "3" give yourself 3 points, "4" give yourself 2 points, and "5" give yourself 1 point. The closer you scored to 50, the more you cherish the quality of competence.

---

and to build competence in a number of ways. For example, the standards stress the necessity for helpers to (1) know the limit and scope of their abilities, (2) seek appropriate consultation when necessary, (3) be involved in ongoing professional development activities, and (4) continually seek out new and better treatment methods. The legal system reinforces these ethical guidelines by noting that helpers "commit professional malpractice if they are visibly less competent than the average of their peers. . . . A function of lawsuits is to encourage competent therapy" (Swenson, 1997, p. 166).

How much do you value the acquisition of knowledge and the importance of being competent? Take the questionnaire in Exercise 1.8 to get a sense of how to rate your competence.

BRINGING IT ALL TOGETHER

This chapter examined eight characteristics that seem to be either empirically or theoretically related to effectiveness as a helper: (1) being empathic, (2) being open, (3) being real, (4) having high internality, (5) being an experiencer of life, (6) having good emotional health, (7) being an alliance builder, (8) being competent. These qualities represent personal characteristics human service professionals should strive to develop. Few if any of us are "already

---

EXERCISE 1.9   Rating My Characteristics

Using the rating scale below, place the appropriate number next to each characteristic based on the importance that *you* place on it, having read this chapter (you may not believe some of the characteristics are as important as I believe they are). Then, using the same rating scale, rate yourself on each characteristic. After you have finished, find two or three persons you believe have gotten to know you well and ask each of them to rate you. In the spaces provided make a note of when, if at all, you exhibited that quality today and what you can do to enhance that characteristic. Completion of this task should give you an overview of how well you display each of the eight characteristics.

When rating, use the scale below. A high rating (closer to "9") indicates that you embody the characteristic, believe it is important, or exhibited the particular characteristic today.

1. An extremely low rating
2. A very low rating
3. A moderately low rating
4. A somewhat low rating
5. Neither high nor low

6. A somewhat high rating
7. A moderately high rating
8. A very high rating
9. An extremely high rating

SELF-INVENTORY

	Importance	Self-Rating	Other Rating	Exhibit Today?	What You Can Do to Improve Scores
Being empathic					
Being open					
Being real					
Having high internality					
Being an experiencer of life					
Having good emotional health					
Being an alliance builder					
Being competent					

there." More likely, each of these qualities should be viewed as road signs as we travel our own unique paths through life. Eventually, as we gain a little more knowledge than before, we may even feel greater comfort just traveling the road. The following exercise (Exercise 1.9) gives you an opportunity to review all the characteristics examined in the chapter.

SUMMARY

This chapter examined the characteristics of the effective helper, those that are important in building a successful helping relationship. Highlighted first was the importance of being empathic—the professional's ability to understand another person's experience of the world. Next was the quality of openness; people with this characteristic are open to criticism, change, and hearing the opinions of others. These individuals readily accept differences in others.

Being real was the next quality explored. Being real, or genuine means living a life that is open, not fake, not deceptive. Individuals who embody this quality are consistent in their feelings, thoughts, and behaviors and are experienced by others as being truthful and transparent.

Being internally oriented was the fourth quality examined. Individuals who are internally oriented take responsibility for their actions and rely more on themselves than on others when making important life decisions. Helpers were cautioned, however, that this characteristic may vary among cultures. Individuals in Western societies tend to value an internal locus of control and an internal locus of responsibility, and these may be culturally specific qualities.

The fifth quality reviewed was being an experiencer of life. People with this characteristic take time to experience and appreciate the world. They are willing to "go with the flow" and be in the moment with their clients. They realize that change occurs slowly and strive to not push clients too fast; instead, they can move with the pace of the client.

The next quality was good emotional health, as the mental health of the helper has been shown to be related to client outcomes. Discussed here was the importance for helpers of experiencing counseling themselves or having some other experience that can improve the quality of their lives.

Alliance building, the seventh quality, has gained some prominence in the literature recently. Helpers can build alliances with clients in many different ways, but regardless of the way these connections are made, the ability to "join" with one's client is important for positive client outcomes.

The last quality explored was competence. One can be competent in many ways, but generally the professional who is competent has a "thirst for knowledge," wants to be involved with his or her professional associations, reads journals, and learns about new techniques.

Finally, we noted these are qualities that human service professionals strive to enhance throughout life; being aware of these characteristics and understanding how they can add to the client–helper relationship can lead to a richer, more rewarding experience as a helper.

INFOTRAC COLLEGE EDITION

Note: Keywords are in quotation marks.

1. Search for information about the effect of "counselor characteristics" on the helping relationship. What characteristics, other than the ones in this chapter, are shown to be important in the helping relationship?

2. Take any one of the eight characteristics listed in this chapter and search for additional information about it.

2

Entering the Agency

INTRODUCTION

When a client initially enters an agency, he or she is immediately faced with aspects of the agency that will either encourage or inhibit openness. The tone is set by how the client experiences the agency during the initial contact, how the client is affected by the atmosphere of the helper's office, and the effect that nonverbal behaviors have on the client, including such things as the helper's attire, eye contact, body positioning and facial expressions, personal space, touch, voice intonation, and tone of voice. These are all examined here. The chapter concludes with a brief discussion of the importance of cross-cultural awareness when considering nonverbal behavior.

CLIENT'S INITIAL CONTACT WITH AGENCY

Generally, clients initially contact agencies by telephoning or by walking in. How an agency initially responds to the client immediately creates a framework for how the client believes he or she will be treated. Thus, agencies need to be particularly cognizant of how clients are cared for during this initial encounter.

Telephone Contact

If a client initially telephones an agency, a number of general guidelines should be followed to help the client feel at ease:

- The agency employee who answers the phone needs to be courteous.

- Agency staff should caringly find out to whom they are talking and what the client is requesting.

- The process for seeing a helper should be explained to the potential client.

- A client who has mistakenly called the wrong agency, which happens quite frequently, should be courteously given available referrals.

- Although a client should not be counseled on the phone (unless this is the type of agency that deals with crisis phone calls), he or she should be assured that there will be an opportunity to talk with a helper when he or she comes to the agency.

- An appointment should be made for the client. If the agency schedule is full and the appointment is several days or weeks in the future, the client should be assessed to ensure that he or she can safely wait that long. If for any reason the client is suspected to need immediate attention (e.g., the client is suicidal), there should be a process to meet his or her needs.

- The client's phone number and/or address should be secured so that he or she can be reminded of the appointment and/or contacted if he or she should fail to come in.

Unfortunately, too often I have been at agencies where the initial phone contact is handled poorly. For instance, I have heard agency staff answer phones using a nasty tone, other staff not obtaining necessary information, and personnel not informing clients of agency procedures. Exercise 2.1 gives students an opportunity to role-play a client's initial telephone call.

EXERCISE 2.1   Telephoning an Agency

Pair up with another student. One of you role-play a client, the other a receptionist responding to the client's phone call. The client should have a reason for contacting the agency. The receptionist should be prepared to respond using the seven points listed above. When you have finished, discuss the exercise in small groups or as a class.

Walking into an Agency

Imagine a client just walking into an agency. She steps into the waiting room and sees a dirty floor and smoked-filled room. There is poor lighting and a bad odor. She walks up to the receptionist, who does not pay attention to her. She says to the receptionist, "Excuse me," and the receptionist looks up and responds, in a rather nasty voice, "What do you want?" and then asks her to sit down and "Wait your turn." She sits down on an old couch and can practically feel the dirt rub off on her skin as her arms touch the armrest.

Now, imagine another agency. A client walks in and notices that the agency smells clean and looks pleasant. A receptionist immediately calls out to him, "I'm sorry that I'm kind of busy at the moment, but I want to talk with you as soon as I can. Please have a seat and I'll be right with you." He says "Thank you" and sits down; although the couch is not new, he can tell that it is clean, and it feels comfortable.

The two vignettes above are real. I've certainly been in agencies where I've had the unfortunate experience represented in the first vignette, as well as the pleasant experience in the second one. As you would guess, the first entry into an agency often leaves a lasting impression on the client and can result in the client's responding in a negative or in a positive fashion to the helper.

I have found that helpers often feel little responsibility for the atmosphere of the agency. I believe that the helping relationship does not start in the helper's office, but with the initial contact the client has with the agency, whether by phone or by walking in. Thus, I encourage all human service professionals to take an active role in creating an agency environment that is conducive to establishing a positive helping relationship. Taking responsibility for the total atmosphere of the agency is also our ethical obligation:

> Human service professionals respect the integrity and welfare of the client at all times. Each client is treated with respect, acceptance and dignity. (Statement 2 of the *Ethical Standards of Human Services Professionals,* see Appendix B.)

> Human service professionals participate in efforts to establish and maintain employment conditions which are conducive to high quality client services. (Statement 33 of the *Ethical Standards of Human Services Professionals,* see Appendix B.)

Many items contribute to creating an inviting atmosphere for clients (e.g., soft lighting, comfortable furniture, placement of furniture), and I am confident that you can come up with a number of items on your own. In class, complete Exercise 2.2, and your instructor will lead a discussion addressing agency atmosphere. When you have completed Exercise 2.2, do Exercise 2.3.

EXERCISE 2.2   Listing Items That Are a Comfort to Clients

List items that, if you were a client walking into an agency, you would like to see that would help you feel more comfortable at that agency. In class, your instructor will make a larger list from the items you offer.

1. _____
2. _____
3. _____
4. _____
5. _____
6. _____
7. _____
8. _____
9. _____
10. _____

EXERCISE 2.3   The Agency Atmosphere: Vignettes

On your own, respond to the following scenarios. Then, in small groups or as a class, discuss your responses.

1. You're a mental health aide at a mental health center. You walk into your agency in the morning and hear the receptionist berating a client. What do you do?
2. You work as a counselor at a group home for the mentally retarded. Despite constant pleas to your advisory board to spend a little money to paint the home and buy some new furniture, they refuse. You are embarrassed when other professionals come to the home to consult with you. What do you do?
3. You realize that most of the staff at your agency do not seem to care that the reception area is dirty and overcrowded. What do you do?

OFFICE ATMOSPHERE

Building a trusting relationship begins with a client's initial contact with the agency, whatever the setting, so offering a space that is quiet, comfortable, and safe, and where confidentiality can be assured is crucial. Often this is the helper's office; even if one is not working out of a formal office, finding a space that offers these qualities is still critical.

EXERCISE 2.4   Arranging Your Office

Take out a blank piece of paper and draw your own office. For furniture, use the suggested items below and place as many (or as few) in your office as you would like (duplicates are allowed). Feel free to add your own pieces of furniture or not to use mine. Compare your office to the office of other students. What makes your office more or less supportive of a positive helping relationship than another student's? Justify your office arrangement based on your counseling style.

Desk	File cabinet	Couch
Chair	Computer	Plant
Bookcase	Coffee table	Sound equipment (e.g., radio, CD player)
End tables	Printer	Pictures
Large lamp	Small lamp	Rocking chair
Desk chair	Wicker basket	Magazine rack

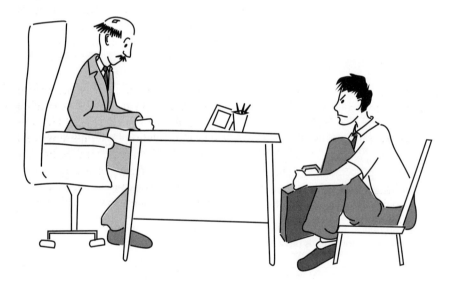

How a helper arranges his or her office can be important in eliciting positive attitudes from clients (Gutheil, 1991; Proshansky, Ittleson, & Rivlin, 1970). Most agree that an office should be relatively soundproof, have soft lighting, be uncluttered, have client records filed, be free from distractions such as the phone ringing or knocks on the door, and have comfortable seating. Large pieces of furniture, like a desk, should generally not be between the helper and the client, although this might vary as a function of the helper's counseling style, personality, and the particular situation (e.g., I've worked with volatile clients when I felt it would be "wise" to have a desk between me and them). As the helper "creates" his or her office, each will try to find a bal-

---

EXERCISE 2.5   Selecting Items to Place in Your Office

Review the items below and decide whether any of them would be offensive to you if you walked into a helper's office. Then think about the most liberal and the most conservative person you know, and imagine how he or she might feel with each of the following:

- Feminist literature
- A bear rug
- Gay literature
- A cluttered desk
- Information on abortion
- Leather furniture
- A Confederate flag

- Fundamentalist religious literature
- A compulsively clean desk
- An AIDS pin
- A desk between you and your client
- Information on female and male sexuality
- A cross
- An American flag

---

ance between having the office reflect his or her taste and having it still be appealing to the vast majority of clients (see Exercise 2.4).

How the helper arranges furniture is not the only thing that will affect whether a client will be open or closed during an interview. Often, the kinds of literature or the type of motif the helper has in his or her office can greatly affect a client's willingness to be open. To highlight this point, complete Exercise 2.5 and then discuss in class whether you think the items listed should be included in one's office.

Of course, no matter how a helper arranges his or her office, some people will be offended by something. Perhaps in deciding how to arrange *your* office you can take a little bit of advice from Scissons (1993) who says, "[A]t the very least, [office] arrangements should not adversely impinge on the process or outcome" of the helping relationship (p. 149). Of course, it may be that you will want to attract certain clientele who would feel comfortable with a particular ambiance. For instance, a Christian counselor might include articles of a religious nature in his or her office, while a person dealing with mostly gay issues might include gay literature.

NONVERBAL BEHAVIOR

Yet when humans communicate, as much as eighty percent of the meaning of their messages is derived from nonverbal language. The implication is disturbing. As far as communication is concerned, human beings spend most of their time studying the wrong thing. (Thompson, 1973, p. 1)

Although nonverbal behaviors span the life of the helping relationship, they will have an immediate effect on how the client initially experiences the helper. The importance of the helper's nonverbal interactions with clients is vastly underrated. In fact, nonverbal behavior seems largely out of a person's conscious control (Argyle, 1975; Wolfgang, 1985), is difficult to censor, and compared to verbal behavior, is often a more accurate representation of how the client and the helper feel (Mehrabian, 1972). Such things as dress, eye contact, posture, and/or tone of voice that communicate "don't open up to me" will obviously affect clients very differently from verbally communicating "I'm open to hearing what you have to say."

Attire

How the helper dresses is an important aspect of a client's initial perception of the helper and can be inviting to a client or can turn a client off. Should jeans be worn at work? What about an expensive suit? Are the helper's clothes revealing? What does jewelry or hair style say about the helper? Are shoes nicely polished or scuffed? Are sneakers okay to wear? Are clothes tucked in neatly, or falling out all over the place? Is it okay to have a pierced nose, eyebrow, or tongue?

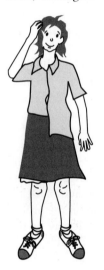 Human service professionals should be very conscious of two factors that should influence the way they dress for work. The first is how their appearance will affect clients. Is there anything in the helper's style of dressing that a client would find offensive or startling? Helpers should learn to consciously consider the client's reactions to their appearance, remembering that how the client perceives them is part of the helpful environment they are trying to create.

The second factor is the agency's dress code—whether this is covert or overt. If the agency has a written dress code, helpers should certainly observe it. Sometimes there are no written rules, but agency employees have established a de facto code in their similarity of dress. If most people in the agency wear jackets, ties, and business suits, a helper would appear out of place in jeans, and this difference would be noticed by clients. The important point is for helpers to realize that what they wear sends a message to clients and to decide what they want that message to be. To help

---

EXERCISE 2.6   Initial Impressions

Get together with three students in your class whom you don't know at all, or at least don't know well. Then, without revealing your name, on a separate piece of blank paper write down your initial impressions of each of the other three students in your group based on what they are wearing. Try to be honest. After you have finished, each person in the group should collect the pieces of paper that represent the responses for himself or herself and read them aloud in the group. While reading the responses, give your reactions to what the group members wrote. Did they seem to accurately represent how you see yourself? If not, why not?

you learn the importance of initial impressions and how they can be affected by appearance, do Exercise 2.6.

Eye Contact

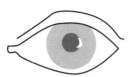

How a helper looks at a client reveals much about the helper's willingness and desire to work with the individual. Similarly, the type of eye contact the client gives the helper can reveal much about the willingness of the client to work with the helper, or potential fears of relating the client may have. Although intense eye contact, such as staring, will certainly turn off almost any client, the helper who has difficulty maintaining any eye contact will not have an easy time building a trusting relationship with a client. Thus, finding the "correct" amount of eye contact that tells a client the helper is ready to listen to him or her is the goal of any helping relationship. For many helpers this comes naturally; however, some helpers have difficulty maintaining eye contact with individuals. You may want to explore your ability to maintain eye contact. Exercise 2.9 explores several nonverbal cues, of which eye contact is one.

Body Positioning and Facial Expressions

One of the most important nonverbal behaviors that clients initially observe is how the helper positions his or her body during the helping relationship. Body posture can telegraph to a client whether the helper wants to work with the client. Does the helper sit with his or her legs crossed? Leaning forward? With arms folded? Researchers of body posture and its messages suggest that optimally, the helper should have his or her feet on the ground, body leaning forward slightly, and arms positioned in a manner that suggests to the client that the helper is ready to listen.

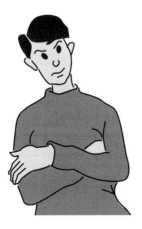

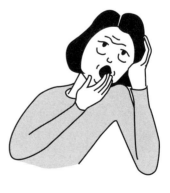

EXERCISE 2.7   Playing with Body Positions

Here's a fun exercise you may have done before. Sit back to back with a partner. One person describes a figure (e.g., a car) while the other person draws it. However, you must not use any words to give away what it is (e.g., tires, steering wheel). For instance, you might say: "Draw a rectangle. Now, place four circles on the bottom of it—two in the front and two in the back." And so forth. Then do the same exercise using a different object but this time facing one another; the person doing the describing needs to keep his or her arms crossed. Then do it one last time, this time using your arms. Reflect on how much easier these activities are when we are able to use our body.

In addition to how the helper positions his or her body, head motions and facial expressions are also very important to the client's experience of the helping relationship. Is the helper's head movement saying to the client, "Yes, I hear you" and "Keep on talking," or is it indicating to the client that the helper is bored, restless, and/or simply not interested? Do the helper's facial expressions show care and concern or does the helper sit with a smirk that says "I don't believe a word you are saying"? In general, body language, through the ways that one positions oneself, as well as facial expressions, are vital communication pieces to the helping relationship. To see how important body language can be, do Exercise 2.7.

Personal Space

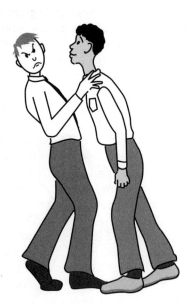

The amount of space between a helper and client is an immediate message to the client about the helping relationship and will positively or negatively affect the relationship (Germain, 1981; Sommer, 1959). Personal space is mediated to some degree by culture, age, and gender, and individuals vary greatly in their level of comfort with personal space (Evans & Howard, 1973). Therefore, the helper must allow for enough personal space that the client feels comfortable, yet not so much that the client feels distant from the helper. Although this will generally happen in very subtle ways, the helper should take the lead in creating an appropriate distance through respect for the client's needs and through

---

EXERCISE 2.8   Personal Space

Here is a quick exercise you can do in class to examine the amount of personal space that feels comfortable to each student in class. Your instructor will have you stand in two lines, with each person facing another person in the class. The two lines should be about five feet apart. The instructor will then request all the students in one line to move a comfortable distance closer to or further away from the students in the other line whom they are directly facing. Based on personal space needs, some students will move closer than others. Then after standing for about fifteen seconds, the students in the other line will be asked to move forward or backward, based on how comfortable they feel with the level of distance between them and the students in the other line. After you have completed standing in your lines, discuss the level of comfort you felt when the person across from you moved closer to or further away from you. What does this say about your comfort with personal space? How do you think this applies to a client's comfort level with personal space?

---

awareness of what might be optimal for the helping relationship. Exercise 2.8 can help you determine your own comfort level regarding personal space.

Touch

Touch is another aspect of nonverbal behavior important to the client's experience of the helping relationship. Of course, touching at important moments is quite natural. For instance, when someone is expressing deep pain, it is not unusual to hold the person's hand, or to embrace the person while he or she sobs. Or, when a person is coming to or leaving a session, many helpers may find it natural to place a hand on a shoulder or give a hug. However, in today's litigious society, touch has become such a delicate subject that it is important for all helpers to be sensitive to their clients' boundaries, their own boundaries, and the limits of touch as suggested by our profes-

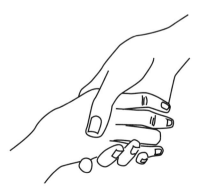

sional ethics (Gabbard, 1995). Some have become so "touchy" over this issue that a therapist in Massachusetts, branded "the hugging therapist," was fired from his job at a mental health agency because he hugged his clients too much. Brammer and MacDonald (1998) suggest that whether one has physical contact with a client should be based on (1) the helper's assessment of the helpee, (2) the helper's awareness of his or her own needs, (3) what

EXERCISE 2.9   Playing with Nonverbal Cues

In class, find a partner and have one person role-play a client discussing a situation of his or her choice. The other person should attempt to listen to the "client" while offering very little eye contact. Then do the same role-play and offer too much eye contact. Then switch roles, having the other person in the dyad role-play a client. You may want to continue this exercise trying to exaggerate or minimize other nonverbal cues such as head nodding, saying "uh huh," touching your client, and so forth. After you have finished the role-play, discuss in class the level of comfort you felt with the various types of nonverbal behaviors you expressed and received.

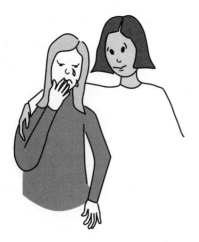

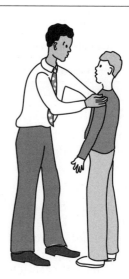

is most likely to be helpful within the helping relationship, and (4) risks that may be involved as a function of agency policy, customs, personal ethics, and the law (see Exercise 2.9).

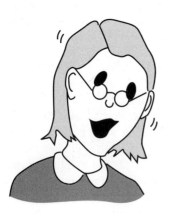

Voice Intonation and Tone

Voice intonation and tone of voice, the final nonverbal aspects of the helping relationship to be explored, can also affect the client's experience of the helper. Helpers must be aware that what they say may not always match how they're saying it. For instance, saying "I like you" in an angry tone, at best, gives a mixed message. Thus, helpers must be keenly aware of what they are communicating through their tone of voice. Also, all helpers will make a number of guttural responses to clients during a session. Such responses as "uh huh" can go a

---

EXERCISE 2.10   Assessing Nonverbal Behavior

In class, break up into groups of five students. Have each student, one at a time, role-play a helper with another student for three or four minutes. The other three students are to watch the role-play, and using the chart below, write comments about the nonverbal behaviors of the student role-playing the helper. After you finish each role-play, give the helper the feedback sheets and discuss what was written.

	Positive Nonverbals	Negative Nonverbals
Attire		
Eye Contact		
Body Language		
Personal Space		
Touch		
Voice Intonation and Tone		

---

long way in telling clients whether they are being attended to. Human communication takes place in many complex ways, more ways than sometimes we would like to admit, and the helper's manner of response can mean more than it seems to mean on the surface (Watzlawick, 1967).

A Cross-Cultural Perspective on Nonverbal Behavior

Traditionally, helpers have been taught to lean forward, have good eye contact, speak in a voice that meets the client's affect, and to rarely touch the client. However, research suggests that there are cross-cultural differences in the ways that clients perceive and respond to such nonverbal helper behaviors (Morse & Ivey, 1996; Sue & Sue, 1990). Therefore, it is now suggested that helpers be acutely sensitive to client nonverbal differences while being knowledgeable and skilled in culturally appropriate responses.

> Culturally skilled helpers are able to engage in a variety of verbal and nonverbal helping responses. They are able to *send* and *receive* both *verbal* and *nonverbal* messages *accurately* and *appropriately.* They are not tied down to only one method or approach to helping but recognize that helping styles and approaches may be culture bound. When they sense that their helping style is limited and potentially inappropriate, they can anticipate and ameliorate its negative impact. (Sue, Arredondo, & McDavis, 1992, p. 483)

Effective cross-cultural helpers must understand that some clients will expect to be looked at, while others will be offended by eye contact; that some clients will expect the helper to lean forward, while others will experience this as an intrusion; and that some clients will expect the helper to touch them, while others will see this as offensive. In respect to nonverbal behavior, effective helpers keep in mind what works for the many, yet are sensitive to what works for the few. The full range of nonverbal communication is explored in Exercise 2.10. How did you do?

SUMMARY

In this chapter a number of items that influence the overall atmosphere of the agency were examined. We looked at how the client experiences the agency during the initial contact, how the client is affected by the atmosphere of the helper's office, and the effect that nonverbal behaviors have on the client, including such things as the helper's attire, eye contact, body positioning and facial expressions, personal space, touch, voice intonation, and tone of voice.

Relative to clients' experience when initially contacting the agency, they generally either call or walk in for their first appointment. Highlighted were ways of making the initial phone contact or walk-in experience feel comfortable for the client.

Next, the physical aspects of an office were discussed: the importance of having the office soundproofed, having soft lighting, assuring that the office is relatively uncluttered, having client records filed, making sure that there are few distractions such as the phone ringing or knocks on the door, and having comfortable seating. Also pointed out were the risks of having items in the office that reflect certain values.

Relative to nonverbal behavior, how the helper dresses can affect his or her ability to form a relationship with the client and the "right" amount of eye contact is crucial to building and maintaining that relationship. Body positioning and facial expressions, personal space, touch, and voice intonation and tone are all ways that helpers communicate with their clients and tell them they are "there for them" or that they don't care about them.

Finally, the chapter concluded with a brief look at cross-cultural issues related to nonverbal behaviors, noting that there are cultural differences in the ways clients respond to nonverbal behaviors. Effective helpers keep in mind that what works for the many is not always helpful and appropriate for all.

INFOTRAC COLLEGE EDITION

1. Examine different aspects of the "office environment" and describe additional characteristics that make an office more supportive for a positive helping relationship.

2. Research the importance of "nonverbal behaviors" within the helping relationship.

SECTION II

Helping Skills

The five chapters in this section focus on the nature of helping skills and provide ample opportunity to practice many of the skills widely used today. The first chapter in the section sets the stage with a model for understanding the relationships among the components of the helping relationship, including theory, helping skills, case conceptualization, and the stages of the helping relationship. The next four chapters provide information of foundational skills, commonly used skills, information-gathering skills, and solution-giving skills—many of the traditional tools of the human service professional.

3

Stages of the Helping Relationship

Theory, Process, and Skills

INTRODUCTION

This chapter is designed to help you understand the complex relationship
among theoretical orientation, conceptualization of client concerns, the stages
of the helping relationship, and the nature of skills in the helping relationship.
The chapter begins with a model to help you understand this relationship.
Next is a discussion of the important of theories as a guide in your work and a
brief overview of five prevalent theories of counseling. Last, the stages of the
helping relationship are described and you have an opportunity to identify attitudes and skills that might be used within each stage.

   As the purpose of this chapter is to help you understand how the application of skills is closely related to the helper's theoretical orientation and knowledge of the stages of the helping relationship, it provides a framework for the
skills described in detail in the next four chapters.

A STAGE MODEL FOR UNDERSTANDING
THE HELPING RELATIONSHIP

There is a rhythm to a helping relationship. If conducted properly by the helper,
the relationship moves forward toward its logical and helpful ending, yet often
the road taken to get there is rocky. Within the helping relationship, all helpers,
regardless of whether they know it, work from some theoretical assumptions. In

other words, every helper has a theory. However, theories are not perfect, and they cannot always predict the direction the relationship will take.

There are stages to the helping relationship. The stages have a predictable order, yet the speed through which they are traveled can vary dramatically, and how fast one transverses them is not always predictable. Also, some skills are more likely than others to be used in certain stages.

The effective helping professional should be cognizant of his or her theory, the stages of the helping relationship, and the skills to be used if that helper is to offer the best opportunity for client growth. Six principles sum up this relationship:

1. The prism through which you see a client is based on your theory of counseling and it affects your understanding of your client.
2. How you understand your client will affect how you conceptualize your client's problems (case conceptualization).
3. This "case conceptualization" will affect the kinds of goals you and your client decide on.
4. How you conceptualize your client will change as you transverse the stages of the helping relationship.
5. The skills you use will change as a function of (1) how you conceptualize your client's concerns, and (2) the stage of the helping relationship in which you find yourself.
6. You must be adept at a number of different skills to effectively apply your theory and respond to changes in the client as you proceed through the stages of the helping relationship.

These six principles show that there is a reciprocal relationship among a helper's theoretical orientation, how the helper conceptualizes his or her clients' problems, the stage of the helping relationship, and the skills the helper uses (see Figure 3.1).

An effective human service professional has learned how to integrate all the techniques that will be learned in this text in a manner that will facilitate client growth. Although techniques will vary as a function of a helper's theoretical orientation, certain techniques are more likely to be found at the beginning stages and others in the later stages of the helping relationship.

USE OF THEORY IN THE HELPING RELATIONSHIP

A counseling theory offers helpers a comprehensive system of counseling and assists the helper in understanding which techniques to apply and how to predict change in clients. Theories are researchable and testable, and they generally come from practice. They provide helpers a way of organizing ideas and lead to suggested plans of actions. Effective helpers must have a theoretical base with which to approach their clients. Otherwise, they would just be

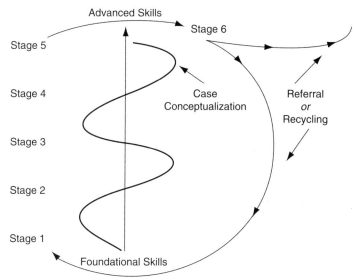

Note: It is assumed that the helper is grounded in theory.

FIGURE 3.1 Relationship Between Case Conceptualization, Theory, Stages, and Skills

"doing their own thing" and there would be no rhyme or reason to client interventions. "To try and function without theory is to operate in chaos, for without placing events in some order it is impossible to function in a meaningful manner" (Hansen, Stevic, & Warner, 1978, p. 16).

This book does not go into detail about theory, within your training program you will almost certainly discuss your theoretical approach to the helping relationship in a class that specifically focuses on theories or in modules that address theory. Understanding the rudiments of theory will help you as you begin to consider why you might choose certain techniques over others. All theory is based on the theorists' view of human nature. Thus, to understand theory, one must understand what is meant by one's view of human nature.

Views of Human Nature as It Relates to Theory

An individual's view of human nature describes how that person understands the reasons people are motivated to do the things they do. For instance, some might believe that behaviors are determined by our genes. Others might believe that behaviors are determined by our environment. Still others might believe that our behaviors are not determined—that we have free will.

The helper's view of human nature affects the kinds of helping skills he or she believes are important. For instance, if a helper's view of human nature is that people are inherently evil, that helper would not want to use

---

**EXERCISE 3.1   The Relationship Between Skills and View
of Human Nature**

On your own, consider which skills you might find useful if your view of human nature was each of the ones listed below. When you have finished with all three, gather in groups of four or five and discuss what you wrote down. Small groups might want to share their findings with the class.

1. You believe that people are born evil and need to control their evil intentions.
2. You believe that there is a natural goodness in people, and they need to learn how to "get in touch" with it.
3. You believe that all behavior is biochemical and the only control we have over our behavior is through changing our biochemistry.

---

skills that lead clients to "be all that they can be." Instead, he or she would probably use skills that assisted individuals to learn how to place restraints on certain aspects of their behavior. Such a helper would want to assist clients in finding ways to control their behavior so their evil would not hurt the world. On the other hand, if a helper believed people are born with innate goodness, that helper would want to use skills that encouraged clients to express their goodness in the world. This helper would want his or her clients to get in touch with their goodness and allow it to blossom (see Exercise 3.1)

There are many items that one can consider when examining one's view of human nature, and you will likely feel more comfortable with the helping skills that are generated from the view of human nature that *you* hold. To examine the things that you believe strongly in, complete Exercise 3.2.

Certain views of human nature lend themselves to specific theoretical approaches to the helping relationship. Following is a very brief summary of the views of human nature underlying five of the more prevalent theoretical approaches. For each of them, consider the view and reflect on whether you share it.

The Views of Human Nature of Five Prevalent
Theories of Counseling

The Psychodynamic Approach Although individuals who adhere to a psychodynamic view may vary considerably on many points, they do share some basic beliefs concerning their view of human nature. For instance, the psychodynamic approach has at its core a belief that drives motivate behavior and that these drives are at least somewhat unconscious. Whereas Freud, who developed the psychoanalytic approach (Corey, 2001), thought that these drives are the instinctual drives of sex and aggression (Appignanesi, 1990; Freud, 1947), other theorists like Alfred Adler (1964) and Erik Erikson (1998)

EXERCISE 3.2   Understanding Your View of Human Nature

For each of the four statements below, circle all items that best describe your view of the person. When you have finished, take all the circled items, and using them as a guide, develop a paragraph describing your view of human nature. (Note: Each statement represents a particular perspective on the view of human nature; that perspective is italicized.) Form small groups of four or five and read your paragraph out loud. Discuss.

1. *Innate.* I believe people are born
   a. good.
   b. bad.
   c. neutral.
   d. with original sin.
   e. restricted by their genetics.
   f. with a growth force which allows them to change throughout life.
   g. capable of being anything they want to be.
   h. with sexual drives that consciously and unconsciously affect their lives.
   i. with aggressive drives that consciously and unconsciously affect their lives.
   j. with social drives that consciously and unconsciously affect their lives.
   k. other attributes? _____

2. *The Developing Person.* Personality development is most influenced by
   a. genetics.
   b. learning.
   c. early child-rearing patterns.
   d. drives.
   e. values that we are taught.
   f. environment.
   g. relationships with others.
   h. biology.
   i. conscious decisions.
   j. unconsciousness.
   k. instincts.
   l. modeling the behavior of others.
   m. relationships we form.
   n. developmental issues (e.g., puberty).
   o. other.

3. *The Change Process.* As a people grow older, I believe they are
   a. capable of major changes in their personality.
   b. capable of moderate changes in their personality.
   c. capable of minor changes in their personality.
   d. incapable of change in their personality.
   e. determined by their early childhood experiences.
   f. determined by their genetics.
   g. determined by how they were conditioned and reinforced.
   h. determined by unconscious motivations.
   i. able to transcend or go beyond early childhood experiences.

4. *How Change Occurs.* Change is likely to be most facilitated by a focus on
   a. the conscious mind.
   b. the unconscious mind.
   c. thoughts.
   d. behaviors.
   e. feelings.
   f. early experiences.
   g. biology.
   h. the past.
   i. the present.
   j. the future.
   k. biology (e.g., the use of medications).
   l. unfinished business and repressed memories.
   m. getting in touch with the "true" self.
   n. other.

believed that people are motivated more by social drives. Still others, such as Heinz Kohut (1984), play down the effects of sex, aggression, and social drives but highlight the ways in which people attach and separate from important "others." And theorists like Carl Jung (1968, 1975) believed that people are motivated by positive unconscious forces that drive them to understand themselves and their relationships to others. Regardless of which motivating force an individual believes is most important, psychodynamically oriented individuals believe that the perceptions of childhood as well as the actual events that occurred during childhood, in combination with drives, greatly affect one's psyche and, consequently, one's later adult development. Therefore, the purpose of psychodynamic therapy is to help the individual understand his or her early childhood experiences and how those experiences, in combination with the individual's drives, motivate the person today.

The Behavioral Approach The behaviorist believes that all behavior is learned and that people are conditioned by reinforcers in their environment. This view does not stress the unconscious and does not place emphasis on gaining insight into early childhood experiences. Instead, this approach assumes that individuals have learned their current behaviors and that they can learn new behaviors by applying the principles of behaviorism. Therefore, the past is not particularly important in the behavioral approach (Corey, 2001).

Because this approach is focused on identifying and changing behaviors, whether using the classical conditioning of Pavlov, the operant conditioning approach of Skinner, or the social-learning or modeling approach of Bandura, all agree that the helper can apply this theory in a straightforward, sometimes technical, manner (Corey, 2001; Neukrug, 1999a). In its early days, the behavioral approach was seen as a directive approach to working with a client in that the client's situation was examined and diagnosed and strategies for behavior change were identified. However, establishing a relationship through such nondirective approaches as the use of empathy and modeling, prior to suggesting specific behavior changes, has recently become more important (Spiegler & Gaeuremont, 1998).

The Humanistic Approach Besides being a reaction to psychodynamic and behavioral theory, the humanistic approach had its origins in existential philosophy and phenomenology (Corey, 2001; Neukrug, 1999a). Therefore, adherents of the humanistic approach believe that people have choices and that they are constantly making choices that shape their existence or way of being in the world. Humanistic approaches, such as those applied through Rogerian counseling or Gestalt therapy, assert that there is no such thing as an objective reality; instead, they stress the subjective reality of the individual. Trying to understand how the individual constructs his or her reality and helping the individual to understand his or her experience of the world is the major goal of this approach. In addition, humanistic theorists generally agree that people are born with some type of actualizing tendency, or growth force. This means that individuals have the ability to transcend their current existence and move toward a more fulfilling and harmonious existence. Therefore, humanists believe that although the past may have been important in affecting how a person acts today, a helping relationship does not have to focus on the past to help a person change and grow.

The Cognitive Approach Cognitive-oriented theorists, such as Albert Ellis and Aaron Beck, tend to believe that the individual's thinking is conditioned starting in early childhood, that one's way of thinking is reinforced throughout one's lifetime, and that how one thinks is directly related to how one acts and feels (Corey, 2001; Neukrug, 1999a). They believe that people are not born with innate goodness or evil, as rational or irrational beings, or as individuals who are depressed, happy, angry, or content. Instead, they believe that people are born neutral. Adherents to the cognitive approach propose that thinking can be changed through counterconditioning; that is, people can reinforce new, healthier ways of thinking. Therefore, what they had learned in childhood can be relearned. Cognitive theorists believe that understanding *why* people behave is not crucial, and perhaps not even important, to making changes in the way they think and act. Such changes in thinking, according to these theorists, will ultimately help clients cope with daily living and will change dysfunctional behavior patterns.

Brief Approaches Human service professionals are generally not practicing in-depth therapy, and they tend to work on very focused problems. For these reasons, brief treatment approaches, which recently have gained tremendously in popularity, are becoming more common with them. Although a person practicing brief approaches to the helping relationship can come from any theoretical background and therefore hold any of a number of different views of human nature, there are some common practices for individuals who are involved in brief approaches. For instance, Garfield (1989) states that they tend to (1) seek practical, pragmatic ways to alleviate problems; (2) view problems as a natural part of life; (3) emphasize a person's strengths; (4) underscore and focus on presenting problems; (5) believe that change can occur after treatment ends; and (6) believe that being in counseling for long periods of time is not necessary for change to occur.

This overview of theoretical perspectives is very brief because an in-depth examination of counseling theories is not a primary goal of this book. However, it should give you an idea of the essential beliefs underlying these five approaches. Now, do Exercise 3.3 to see where your views fit among the five theories.

EXERCISE 3.3   Your View of Human Nature and Theoretical Approach

To the left of each statement listed below, place the appropriate number. Then when you have finished, follow the directions for scoring the inventory.

> 0 = I do not believe this is true
> 1 = I mildly believe this is true
> 2 = I strongly believe this is true
> 3 = I very strongly believe this is true

1. ____ People can go beyond their early childhood experiences and make major personality changes in their lives.
2. ____ Counseling can take place in a relatively short period of time.
3. ____ People are born with a self-actualizing tendency, but due to experiences they may lose touch with their goodness. However, if they are placed in a nurturing environment, their goodness will generally reemerge.
4. ____ Reinforcements in the environment greatly affect how we act.
5. ____ We are born with drives that greatly affect how we live our lives. Often these drives are out of our consciousness; that is, we behave in ways to get our drives met yet we don't realize that this is the underlying reason for why we're doing what we're doing.
6. ____ My sexual urges greatly affect my behavior in mysterious and unknown ways.
7. ____ My thinking affects my feelings.
8. ____ My behaviors affect my feelings.
9. ____ I have a number of instincts that may affect my behavior in mysterious and known ways.
10. ____ Although some change is possible, much of my life is predestined due to my early childhood experiences.
11. ____ I know that if I can change the way I perceive the world and the way I think, I can live a well-adjusted life.
12. ____ Understanding a client's personality formation from a critical and objective standpoint is probably the most crucial factor in helping a client manage his or her problems.
13. ____ Long-term counseling is relatively a waste of time and money as the same kinds of changes can take place in a brief amount of time.
14. ____ My early childhood may have affected me greatly, but it does not determine my present-day behavior.
15. ____ My early childhood affected me greatly and continues to affect how I live; there is only a limited amount of control I have to change my life.
16. ____ Unconditional positive regard is an essential element in the counseling relationship.
17. ____ We have the ability of controlling the environment for a person and therefore allowing the person to feel good about who he or she is.
18. ____ It is not events that cause me to feel badly; it is what I believe about those events.
19. ____ The bottom line is that things outside of me greatly control my life; I have little ability to change how I feel about myself if events around me are horrible.
20. ____ The change process should be focused on the future, not on current problems.

21.____ How I act is the major force in creating my mental health.
22.____ How I feel is the major force in creating my mental health.
23.____ My behavior affects my thinking.
24.____ I believe that the most crucial aspect for effective helping is the relationship between the helper and client.
25.____ I am in control of most of my behaviors.
26.____ My unconscious controls most of my behaviors.
27.____ My early childhood probably affected my way of thinking, but I can change the way I think and live a healthier life.
28.____ A positive attitude toward life and belief in the ability of people to change is the most crucial aspect in working to help a client work through his or her problems.
29.____ How we make meaning in the world is complex and can best be understood through the stories clients tell.
30.____ Probably, long-lasting change is more affected by my ability to "catch" and change my "automatic" thoughts.
31.____ It is important that I maintain certain defenses in order to live reasonably in this world.
32.____ I believe that the *most* crucial aspect of the counseling relationship is the ability to be empathic with the client.
33.____ My theoretical orientation is not as important as my ability to help the client focus on the future and his or her change process.
34.____ My feelings affect my behavior and cognitions.
35.____ If placed in a nurturing environment, I will be able to get in touch with my "true" self.
36.____ If we can understand the types of parenting that occurred through predictable stages of child development, we can understand the problem of living faced by individuals later in life.

Scoring the Inventory: For each item on the inventory listed below, place the number that you gave that item on your inventory. For instance, if you placed a "3" under item "5," a "3" should be written under the first item under "psychodynamic." Note that some items are used for more than one approach (e.g., item number "1" is used for humanistic, behavioral, cognitive, and brief approaches). When you have finished placing all of the numbers in the appropriate spaces, add up your scores. Because there are fewer items for "Brief/Solution Focused Counseling," you need to multiply your results by a correction factor of 1.4. Note that some might differ with my categorization of items on the inventory. However, your results should give you an approximation of the theoretical orientation toward which you lean.

Psychodynamic	Humanistic	Behavioral	Cognitive	Brief/Solution Focused
5 ___ =	1 ___ =	1 ___ =	1 ___ =	1 ___ =
6 ___ =	2 ___ =	2 ___ =	2 ___ =	2 ___ =
9 ___ =	3 ___ =	4 ___ =	7 ___ =	13 ___ =
10 ___ =	14 ___ =	8 ___ =	11 ___ =	14 ___ =
12 ___ =	16 ___ =	13 ___ =	13 ___ =	20 ___ =
15 ___ =	22 ___ =	14 ___ =	14 ___ =	28 ___ =
19 ___ =	24 ___ =	17 ___ =	18 ___ =	33 ___ =
26 ___ =	32 ___ =	21 ___ =	27 ___ =	Total =
31 ___ =	34 ___ =	23 ___ =	29 ___ =	Total × 1.4 =
36 ___ =	35 ___ =	25 ___ =	30 ___ =	
Total =	Total =	Total =	Total =	Total =

EXERCISE 3.4   Skills Associated with Each Theoretical Approach

Highlighted below are some major points in the views of human nature of the five approaches we have discussed. Examine each of these lists, and for each theoretical approach, make a list of the skills you believe would be necessary if applying that approach. When that is completed, in the space provided, write in five major points of your view of human nature and then jot down a list of the skills that would be important for you to use. As you read through the text, you might want to pay particular attention to any skills identified that match the ones you highlighted as important to your view of human nature.

Psychodynamic

1. Early childhood experiences
2. Innate drives
3. The unconscious
4. Instincts
5. Sex/aggression, and/or social drives

Humanistic

1. Goodness of person
2. Focus on present
3. Actualizing tendency
4. Growth force
5. Positivistic approach

Behavioral

1. Focus on behaviors
2. Focus on present
3. Conditioned behavior
4. Reinforcements
5. Environment

Cognitive Approach

1. Conditioning is important
2. Thinking affects behavior
3. People are born neutral
4. What is learned can be relearned
5. Past is not really important

Brief Approaches

1. Are pragmatic and practical
2. Problems are natural part of life
3. Emphasize person's strengths
4. Consider presenting problems important
5. Counseling not need be long and change continues after counseling

Your Approach

1. _____

2. _____

3. _____

4. _____

5. _____

Skills Associated with Varying Theories

Because each theory is unique in its view of human nature, the skills that are stressed will vary. Now that you've explored your theoretical orientation as well as your view of human nature, you may want to consider further how each of these can affect the helping relationship. You can do this with Exercise 3.4.

What About the Skills We Will Learn in This Text?
How Do They Fit in All of This?

Although some skills are more specific to certain theories—and there are many skills that are not discussed in this text—most of the skills highlighted in this book tend to be transtheoretical; that is, they are used by most helpers. Thus, almost all theoretical approaches will incorporate the use of the foundational skills of basic listening and empathic responding that are discussed in Chapter 4. In addition, many if not all the theoretical approaches will practice some form of the commonly used skills in Chapter 5, which include affirmation giving, encouragement, self-disclosure, and modeling. The information-gathering skills and helper-centered skills of Chapter 6 and Chapter 7 are more frequently used by behaviorists, cognitive-oriented helpers, and brief treatment helpers; however, helpers from almost all theoretical backgrounds are being increasingly asked to conduct brief treatment, so these skills are now being used more and more frequently by all helpers.

STAGES OF THE HELPING RELATIONSHIP

Because the roles and functions of the human service professional can vary considerably, many different types of interviewing can occur. For instance, some human service professionals may do more information gathering, others may do more supportive work, and others may do mostly counseling. Some may be seeing clients for 15 minutes, others for a couple of hours. Some will see a client one time, others for a few years. However, regardless of the kind of interviewing the helper is doing, there are stages of the helping relationship that all clients and helpers go through. These stages may span one session or may continue over the lifetime of the helping relationship. In either case, the effective helping professional should be cognizant of these stages as the attitudes and skills most appropriate for each of the stages vary. Thus, just as skills vary as a function of one's theory, they also change as a function of the stage of the helping relationship.

The Pre-Interview Process

Prior to actually undertaking the interview there is a pre-interview process that includes everything that happens to the client prior to his or her actually sitting down with the assigned helper. For instance, it is the rare agency today that does not have the client fill out a massive amount of paperwork as soon as he or she enters the door. Regardless of who might be assisting the client in the completion of this task, it is important that the individual is kind, courteous, and thoughtful—even in those cases when the client is not!

In addition to the initial paperwork, increasingly clients will undergo what is called an intake interview soon after coming to the agency. This intake interview is frequently conducted by a helper other than the one who is eventually assigned to the client. Often, it is at this point that a structured interview will take place (see Chapter 6), and it is crucial that this first encounter with the helper is a positive experience for the client, as it can determine the nature of the helping relationship to come. Exercise 3.5 allows you to experience the pre-interview process.

EXERCISE 3.5   The Pre-Interview Process

This exercise can be completed with the whole class or in small groups. The
instructor, or students who have worked at an agency, may want to bring some
samples of paperwork that clients complete when first entering an agency. The
instructor may want to rearrange the classroom so it has more of an agency
waiting room feel. Next, the instructor should identify a fictitious "agency"
which a client will enter. Then, a student will volunteer to role-play a client
who will be assigned to a role-play helper. A role-play secretary should also be
identified. The secretary should discuss with the instructor the process the
client will go through at the agency. The secretary will later explain this process
to the client.

The client will walk into the agency and make initial contact with the
secretary. The secretary will then explain to the client the process he or she will
go through at the agency and give any paperwork that needs to be completed
to the client. When the paperwork is completed, the secretary will refer the
client to a helper to complete any additional paperwork (if you wish, the
helper can use the structured interviewed format as delineated in Box 6.2 on
pages 91–92, to gather information from the client). When the exercise is
complete, answer the following questions (you may want to refer to Chapter 2
when reviewing the questions).

1. Did the client feel comfortable in this agency?
2. Could the client have been treated in a more humane fashion?
3. Was the process effective for gathering preliminary data from the client?
4. Did the client have a feel for what was going to happen to him or her?
5. Are there any other suggestions for making this process better?

Stage 1: Rapport and Trust Building

After completing the necessary forms and perhaps a structured intake interview, the client will be assigned a helper with whom to work. Clients come
to the helper with one major agenda: "Can I trust my helper enough to discuss with him or her what I need to discuss?" The helper, on the other hand,
is dealing with a number of technical issues that are crucial to the development of an effective working relationship. For instance, the helper should be
concerned with assuring that the physical environment feels safe, offering a
professional disclosure statement (a statement describing the nature of the
helping relationship), and obtaining informed consent (consent for the specific kind of treatment to be offered) (Brammer & MacDonald, 1998; Scissons, 1993). (Note: Professional disclosure statements and informed consent
will be discussed in more detail in Chapter 6 and Chapter 10.)

After the technical issues are taken care of, the helper wants to attend to
the primary goal of the first stage—development of a comfortable, trusting,
and facilitative relationship. During these beginning sessions, helpers will often

---

BOX 3.1   Reality Versus Ideal

I have worked in and visited enough agencies to know that the human service professional does not always have the luxury of extended periods of time to build relationships with clients. Often, the job of the human service professional becomes a paperwork shuffle in which he or she is swiftly gathering information and making some rather quick decisions about the future of a client. However, I think it bears keeping in mind that the best human service professionals are those who are able to remember the importance of relationship building when attending to the problems of another human being. I think we must consider what our purpose is if we are doing little more than paper shuffling.

---

discuss superficial items or common interests with clients in an effort to establish a camaraderie. However, the helper does not want to make the session too "chatty" and should remember that although a helper may be friendly with a client, he or she is not the client's friend. The helper should also keep in mind that in addition to building trust, a major purpose of this stage is to facilitate client disclosure of self-identified problems. This is best accomplished by demonstrating through the use of helping skills that the helper understands the client. It is through this understanding that the client will feel safe and trusting enough to open up.

As this stage continues, the helper will begin to identify and eventually delineate the issues presented by the client. The helper should review and evaluate the accuracy of this list with the client by reflecting to the client those problems thought to be highlighted during this stage, or by asking the client directly if the list is accurate. It is also at this time that helpers will begin to make a preliminary diagnostic assessment of the client. This can include a vocational assessment, medical diagnosis, or mental health diagnoses, like the ones that will be discussed in Chapter 8. Before you go to Stage 2, do Exercise 3.6.

Stage 2: Problem Identification

The building of a trusting relationship and the ability to do an assessment of client problems is a sign that the helper and client are moving into the second stage of the helping relationship. The main purpose of this stage is to have the helper and client validate the initial identification of the problem(s). Because initial concerns may be masking other issues, and because other issues may arise as the helper assists the client in clarifying thoughts and feelings and understanding his or her problem in more depth, it is important that this validation take place. Thus, it is during this stage that the helper validates his or her original assessment and diagnosis and/or makes appropriate changes as necessary. Before you go on, do Exercise 3.7.

EXERCISE 3.6   Stage 1 Skills and Attitudes

In small groups consider the kinds of skills or attitudes you think would be critical for the Rapport and Trust-Building Stage. Make a list of them, and share them with the class. The instructor should write them on the board and the class should choose three to six of these skills or attitudes that might seem particularly important for this stage. Lastly, place the three to six skills or attitudes in Box 3.2 near the end of the chapter.

EXERCISE 3.7   Stage 2 Skills and Attitudes

In small groups, consider the kinds of skills or attitudes you think would be critical for the Problem Identification Stage. Make a list of them, and share them with the class. The instructor should write them on the board and the class should choose three to six skills or attitudes that might seem particularly important for this stage. Lastly, place the three to six skills or attitudes in Box 3.2.

EXERCISE 3.8   Stage 3 Skills and Attitudes

In small groups, consider the kinds of skills or attitudes you think would be critical for the Goal-Setting Stage. Make a list of them, and share them with the class. The instructor should write them on the board and the class should choose three to six skills or attitudes that might seem particularly important for this stage. Lastly, place the three to six skills or attitudes in Box 3.2.

Stage 3: Goal Setting

After gathering information and clarifying the client's problems, the helper can work with the client to set some general and/or specific goals. These goals should be based on the information gained thus far in the interview and should be a collaborative process; that is, the helper alone is not setting goals for the client. Instead, it is a joint effort in which the helper and the client determine what goals would best meet the client's needs. In choosing goals with clients, helpers should make sure the goals are an outgrowth of the information obtained in the previous stages and that they are attainable. Do Exercise 3.8.

EXERCISE 3.9   Stage 4 Skills and Attitudes

In small groups, consider the kinds of skills or attitudes you think would be critical for the Work Stage. Make a list of them, and share them with the class. The instructor should write them on the board and the class should choose three to six skills or attitudes that might seem particularly important for this stage. Lastly, place the three to six skills or attitudes in Box 3.2.

EXERCISE 3.10   Stage 5 Skills and Attitudes

In small groups, consider the kinds of skills and attitudes you think would be critical for the Closure Stage. Make a list of them, and share them with the class. The instructor should write them on the board and the class should choose three to six skills or attitudes that might seem particularly important for this stage. Lastly, place the three to six skills or attitudes in Box 3.2.

Stage 4: Work

During this stage, the client is beginning to work on the issues that were identified in Stage 2 and the goals agreed upon between the helper and client in Stage 3. If the Stage 4 skills are used wisely, the helper should be able to increasingly assist the client in facilitating progress toward completion of goals. Of course, if in this process previous goals are clarified or new issues arise, the helper and client may want to reevaluate past goals and even set new ones. Finally, as clients work on goals it is important that the helper affirm and encourage the clients progress. To help crystallize your thinking about stage 4, do Exercise 3.9.

Stage 5: Closure

Whether it comes at the end of the first interview or at the end of the helping relationship, closure is crucial if the client (and helper) are to have a sense of completion. Closure involves summarizing what has been completed, determining whether goals have been met, and discussing how the client feels about the ending of the interview or the helping relationship. During this stage the helper also may wish to discuss his or her feelings about the session or helping relationship coming to the end. For instance, it is not unusual for a helper to say something like, "I feel good about what you discussed today," or "You've spent a few weeks working on some important issues, and I'm proud of what you've done." Now do Exercise 3.10.

EXERCISE 3.11   Stage 6 Skills and Attitudes

In small groups, consider the kinds of skills or attitudes you think would be critical for the Post-Relationship Stage. Make a list of them, and share them with the class. The instructor should write them on the board and the class should choose three to six skills or attitudes that might seem particularly important for this stage. Lastly, place the three to six skills or attitudes in Box 3.2.

Stage 6: The Post-Relationship—The Revolving Door

We believe that patients can and should return as needed" (Budman & Gurman, 1988, p. 20).

The end of the helping relationship may not be the end. Clients may return with new issues, may want to revisit old issues, or may desire to delve deeper into themselves. In fact, it is not unusual for clients to return to the same helper or seek out another helper at some other date (Neukrug & Williams, 1993; Neukrug, 2001). Following up with clients, thus, is crucial in assuring that clients feel satisfied with what they accomplished; it can also act as a check to see whether clients would like to return for additional assistance or be referred to another helper. Follow–up also allows the helper to assess whether change has been maintained.

Follow-up is generally completed a few weeks to six months after the help-ing relationship has ended. This process enables the helper to decide which techniques have been most successful, gives him or her the opportunity to re-inforce past change, and acts as one way in which the helper can evaluate ser-vices provided (Hutchins & Cole, 1992; Kleinke, 1994; Neukrug, 1999a, 2000). Some helpers follow up by a phone call; others send a letter; others do a more elaborate survey of clients. Use Exercise 3.11 to identify your follow-up skills.

SUMMARY OF IDENTIFIED SKILLS AND ATTITUDES OF THE STAGES OF THE HELPING RELATIONSHIP

Use the grid in Box 3.2 to summarize the skills and attitudes identified in pre-vious exercises throughout the chapter.

BOX 3.2 Identified Skills and Attitudes of the Stages of the Helping Relationship

In the space provided, write in the skills and attitudes that were identified by students in the class as being important for each specific stage. The instructor and students may then want to identify the chapter in which these skills will be discussed. Make a note if some identified skills or attitudes are not examined in the text. Consider why they were not. Should they be added? When you finish learning about the skills at the conclusion of Chapter 7, you might want to compare your list to the list in Appendix C.

Note: The characteristics of the effective helper, as noted in Chapter 1, should be in evidence throughout the stages.

Stage	Skills and Attitudes	Chapter
Pre-Interview		
Stage 1: Rapport and Trust-Building		
Stage 2: Problem Identification		
Stage 3: Goal Setting		
Stage 4: Work		
Stage 5: Closure		
Stage 6: Post-Interview: The Revolving Door		

SUMMARY

This chapter began by offering a model for understanding the relationship between theory, case conceptualization, stages of the helping relationship, and the skills used within the helping relationship. This model presented six principles: (1) The prism through which we see our clients is based on our theory of counseling; (2) we conceptualize client problems based on our theory; (3) our case conceptualization affects the goals we choose; (4) as we transverse the stages of the helping relationship, our conceptualization of our client changes; (5) skills used are based on how we conceptualize our client's concerns and on the stage of the helping relationship in which we find ourselves; and (6) you must be adept at many skills to effectively apply your theory and respond to changes in the client as you proceed through the stages of the helping relationship. These principles highlight the complex relationship among theory, the stages of the helping relationship, and the skills that might be used in the various stages.

Theory was discussed briefly, as a helper's view of human nature determines the theoretical orientation to which he or she adheres. The view of human nature underlying five theoretical orientations was examined. The five were psychodynamic, humanistic, behavioral, cognitive, and brief treatment approaches.

Next, the stages of the helping relationship were studied, beginning with the Pre-interview Process in which the client's initial interviews occur. After the client is assigned to work with a professional, he or she enters Stage 1 of the helping relationship, Rapport and Trust Building. The crucial work of this stage is to help the client feel comfortable, understood, and ready to disclose his or her self-identified problems.

Stage 2, Problem Identification, focuses on the helper's initial assessment of the client's problem, validating his or her assessment and diagnosis, and/or making appropriate changes as necessary. After the problems to work on are identified, the helping relationship enters Stage 3, Goal Setting. In this collaborative stage, the helper and client together determine the goals of the helping relationship. In Stage 4, Work, the client focuses on reaching his or her set goals. In Stage 5, Closure, helper and client summarize what has been completed, determine whether goals have been met, and discuss how the client feels about the ending of the helping relationship. As the end is not necessarily the end, clients next move into Stage 6, the Post-stage Process, or the Revolving Door. In this stage, it is important for helpers to follow up with clients—a few weeks to six months later—to assure that all is going well. Follow-up allows the helper to obtain feedback about the maintenance of client progress and to see whether the client needs additional contact with a helper. Throughout the chapter students had the opportunity to identify possible skills and attitudes they thought might be important in each stage of the relationship.

INFOTRAC COLLEGE EDITION

1. Take any one of the theorists within the views of human nature and examine their view and theory in more depth (e.g., Freud, Rogers, Pavlov, Beck).

2. Research the factors in addition to theory that affect one's "case conceptualization."

4

Foundational Skills

INTRODUCTION

The skills in this chapter are considered foundational to any helping relationship because they are essential in establishing the relationship, building rapport and trust, setting a tone with the client, and beginning the client's process of self-examination. Although important throughout the helping relationship, these skills are generally most crucial near the beginning of the relationship and should be continually revisited especially when an impasse is reached. They include the ability to use silence effectively, good listening skills, and showing accurate empathy to clients.

SILENCE AND PAUSE TIME

When	is	empty	space	facilitative,	and	when
does	it	become	a	bit	much?	

Silence is a powerful tool in the helping relationship that can be used advantageously for the growth of the client (Hutchins & Cole, 1992; Kleinke, 1994). It allows the client to reflect on what he or she has been saying. It allows the helper to process the session and to formulate his or her next response. It says to the client that communication does not always have to be filled with words, and it gives the client an opportunity to look at how words can sometimes be used to divert the client from his or her feelings. Silence is

---

EXERCISE 4.1   Silence

Pair up with another student in the class. Have one person role play a helper while the other role plays a client. The client should begin to role play a counseling situation and continue talking for about one minute at which point the instructor should yell out "stop." The helper should then formulate a response to the client but wait until the instructor says "go" to say it. The instructor will wait 30 seconds before saying go, and then the helper should give his or her response. After the helper gives his or her response, discuss how it felt to wait this relatively short amount of time. You may want to do this a few times with different amounts of "pause times," and make sure each student gets to be the helper.

---

powerful. It will sometimes raise anxiety within the client, anxiety that on the one hand could push the client to talk further about a particular topic, and on the other hand could cause a client to drop out of treatment. In short, to be an effective listener, you must be able to maintain a certain amount of silence in the helping relationship, for if you are always filling silent spaces, you are not listening.

I'm sure that after you complete Exercise 4.1, you will agree that 30 seconds is a *very long time* to wait before making a response. Although waiting that long is fairly unusual, you probably found that waiting before responding not only allowed you to formulate your response but also gave the other person an opportunity to think about what he or she said as well as to consider what to say next. You might want to continue the role-play after you have finished Exercise 4.1 to find what amount of silence would feel comfortable to you when making a response *and* facilitate the helping relationship.

Silence on the part of the helper or client may be somewhat culturally determined. For instance, some research has found that the "pause time" for different cultures varies. In fact, Tafoya (1996) notes that Native Americans have at times been labeled reticent to talk and resistant to treatment when in fact the pause time for some Native Americans is longer than for other cultural groups. If they had been treated by Native American helpers, they most likely would not have been labeled in this fashion. Therefore, how people respond to one another will vary as a function of culture. As a helper, you may want to consider your pause time to discover your comfort level with silence while at the same time recognize that your client's pause time might vary as a function of cultural heritage.

LISTENING

First there is the hearing with the ear, which we all know; and the hearing with the non-ear, which is a state like that of a tranquil pond, a lake that is completely quiet and when you drop a stone into it, it makes little waves that disappear. I think that [insight] is the hearing with the non-ear, a state where there is absolute quietness of the mind; and when the question is put into the mind, the response is the wave, the little wave. (Krishnamurti, cited in Jayakar, 1986, p. 325)

How do you listen? Exercise 4.2 will help you find out.

EXERCISE 4.2   Listening Quiz

Take this quiz before you read any further. Next to each item below, place an "X" in the appropriate space to represent how you *generally* respond to someone to whom you are attempting to listen. Then, go through the list again and this time, next to each item, place an "O" to represent how you think you *should* listen to another.

U = Usually   S = Sometimes   R = Rarely

U   S   R

___ ___ ___ 1. I try to determine what should be talked about during the interview.

___ ___ ___ 2. When listening to someone, I prepare myself physically by sitting in a way that I can make sure that I hear what is being said.

___ ___ ___ 3. I try to be "in charge" and lead the conversation.

___ ___ ___ 4. I usually clear my mind and take on a nonjudgmental attitude when listening to another.

___ ___ ___ 5. When listening to another, I try to tell the other my opinion of what he or she is doing.

___ ___ ___ 6. I try to decide from the other's *appearance* whether what he or she is saying is worthwhile.

___ ___ ___ 7. I attempt to ask questions if I need further clarification.

___ ___ ___ 8. I try to judge from the opening statement whether I know what is going to be said.

___ ___ ___ 9. I try to listen intently to feelings.

___ ___ ___ 10. I try to listen intently to content.

___ ___ ___ 11. I try to tell the other person what is "right" about what he or she is saying.

___ ___ ___ 12. I try to "analyze" the situation and give interpretations.

___ ___ ___ 13. I try to use *my* experiences to best understand the other person's feelings.

___ ___ ___ 14. I try to convince the other person the "correct" way to view the situation.

___ ___ ___ 15. I try to have the last word.

Now that you have finished this short quiz, in class or in small groups, use the definition below or come up with your own definition of "listening" and see whether your responses reflect this definition.

Webster asserts that "to listen" means

(1) to pay attention to
(2) to hear something through thoughtful attention: to give consideration
(3) to be alert, to catch an expected sound
(4) to give close attention in order to hear

Although easy to define, listening is one of the most difficult skills to implement as Americans are rarely taught how to hear another person. In fact, ask an untrained adult to listen to another, and usually he or she ends up interrupting and giving advice. Summarizing some of the reasons it is important to be an effective listener, Scissons (1993) stresses that listening helps to build trust, convinces the client that he or she is being understood, encourages the client to reflect on what he or she has just said, ensures the helper that he or she is on the right track, and is an effective way of collecting information from a client without the potentially negative side effects of using questions. (The use of questions is discussed in Chapter 6.)

Hindrances to Effective Listening

Even when we "know" how to listen, a number of factors can prevent us from listening effectively. Work through Exercise 4.3 and explore some of these hindrances to listening in class.

You will likely discover from Exercise 4.3 several potential hindrances to listening. These can have a very negative effect in a helping relationship. Six of these hindrances appear in the following list, expressed in terms of a helper-client interaction:

1. *preconceived notions:* having preconceived notions about the client that interfere with the helper's ability to hear the client

---

EXERCISE 4.3 Hindrances to Listening

In class, break into triads (groups of three). Within your group, each person will take the number 1, 2, or 3. With the three topics listed below (or other topics of the instructor's choice) have the instructor assign one of the topics to persons "1" and "2." Now, number "1" you represent the "pro" side and number "2" you represent the "con" position. One of you start debating the situation while the other "listens." When the first person has finished, the second person should repeat *verbatim* what he or she heard. Then, debate back and forth, taking turns listening and repeating verbatim until the instructor tells you to stop. Number "3," you are an objective "helper," to give feedback if needed. As the objective person, also remember to give feedback concerning each person's body language. When you have finished this first situation, have numbers "2" and "3" do the second situation, and then numbers "3" and "1" do the third situation with the third person being the "objective helper."

When you have finished, the instructor will ask for feedback concerning what things prevented you from hearing the other person. List these "hindrances to listening" on the board. Make sure you discuss some of the following items: preoccupation, defensiveness, emotional blocks, and distractions.

Some Possible Situations: Abortion, Capital Punishment, Gays in the Military, Affirmative Action, National Health Insurance, Welfare Reform, Homosexual Marriages

2. *anticipatory reaction:* anticipating what the client is about to say and not actually hearing the client

3. *cognitive distractions:* thinking about what you are going to say and therefore blocking what the client is saying

4. *personal issues:* having personal issues that interfere with your ability to listen

5. *emotional response:* having a strong emotional reaction to your client's content and therefore not being able to hear the client accurately

6. *distractions:* being distracted by such things as noises, temperature of the office, hunger pains, and so forth

What other hindrances did you discover besides those listed above?

Good Listening

Good listening is intimately related to client outcomes. A good listener

1. talks minimally

2. concentrates on what is being said

3. does not interrupt

4. does not give advice

5. gives and does not expect to get

6. accurately hears the content of what the client is saying

7. accurately hears the feelings in what the client is saying

8. is able to communicate to the client that he or she has been heard (e.g., head nods, uh huhs, reflecting back to the client what the helper heard)

9. asks clarifying questions such as "I didn't hear all of that. Can you explain that in another way so I'm sure I understand you?)"

10. does not ask other kinds of questions

BOX 4.1   Listen to Me

When I ask you to listen to me, and you start giving me advice you have not done what I asked.

When I ask you to listen to me and you begin to tell me why I shouldn't feel that way, you are trampling on my feelings.

When I ask you to listen to me and you feel you have to do something to solve my problem, you have failed me, strange as that may seem.

Listen: All that I ask is that you listen, not talk or do—just hear me.

When you do something for me that I can and need to do for myself, you contribute to my fear and inadequacy.

But when you accept as a simple fact that I do feel what I feel, no matter how irrational, then I can quit trying to convince you and get about this business of understanding what's behind these feelings.

So, please listen and just hear me.

And, if you want to talk, wait a minute for your turn—and I'll listen to you.

(Author Unknown)

Preparing Yourself for Listening

When you are ready to listen, the following practical suggestions should assist you in your ability to hear a client effectively (Egan, 2001; Ivey & Ivey, 1998):

- *Calm yourself down.* Prior to meeting with your client, calm yourself down—meditate, pray, jog, or blow out air, but calm your inner self.
- *Stop talking and don't interrupt.* You cannot listen while you are talking.
- *Show interest.* With your body language and tone of voice, show the person you're interested in what he or she is saying.
- *Don't jump to conclusions.* Take in all of what the person says and don't assume you understand the person more than he or she understands himself or herself.
- *Actively listen.* Many people do not realize that listening is an active process that takes deep concentration. If your mind is wandering, you are not listening.
- *Concentrate on feelings.* Listen, identify, and acknowledge what the person is feeling.
- *Concentrate on content.* Listen, identify, and acknowledge what the person is saying.
- *Maintain appropriate eye contact.* Show the person with your eyes that you are listening, but be sensitive to cultural differences in amount of eye contact given.
- *Have an open body posture.* Face the person and show the person you are ready to listen through your body language, but be sensitive to cultural differences.
- *Be sensitive to the amount of personal space.* Be close enough to the client to show him or her that you are ready to listen, but have a sense of the amount of personal space that is comfortable to your client.
- *Don't ask questions.* Questions are often an indication that you are not listening. Try to avoid questions unless they are clarifying ones (e.g., "Can you tell me more about that?").

Listening comes with practice. Exercise 4.4 is a good beginning point.

EXERCISE 4.4   Practicing Listening Skills

Pair up with two other students in your class in order to practice your listening skills. Have one person role-play a client while the other listens. The third person will be an observer who can give feedback as to how well the listener heard what the "client" said. The listener should first prepare himself or herself for listening as noted above. Then, he or she should make sure that there are as few hindrances to listening as possible. Next, this person should try to listen actively by paraphrasing what his or her partner has said. After the first role-play, have a different student play the client, listener, and observer. Then, do a third role-play giving the last student an opportunity to be the listener.

EMPATHIC UNDERSTANDING

Listed as one of the important helper qualities in Chapter 1, empathy is also an important skill in the helping relationship. Empathy, as an important help-ing skill has been alluded to for centuries (Gompertz, 1960), but it wasn't until the twentieth century that empathy was formally incorporated into the help-ing relationship. Probably the person who has had the greatest impact on our modern understanding and use of empathy is Carl Rogers.

> The state of empathy, or being empathic, is to perceive the internal frame of reference of another with accuracy and with the emotional compo-nents and meanings which pertain thereto as if one were the person, but without ever losing the "as if" condition. (Rogers, 1959, pp. 210–211)

Empathy is the act of showing the client that he or she has been heard. This can be done in many ways, including the use of reflective listening tech-niques; it involves making statements that accurately paraphrase the meaning of what the client has said. However, good empathic responses are much more than what has been popularized as "active or reflective listening." In fact, many master therapists become very creative and mix reflective listening responses with metaphors, analogies, and self-disclosure in an attempt to let the client know that he or she has been heard accurately and his or her feelings have been understood (Neukrug, 1997).

The popularity of Rogers's use of empathy during the twentieth century eventually led to the development of a popular five-point scale to measure empathy. Known as the Carkhuff scale after its developer, this instrument has been widely used in the training of helpers (Gazda, Asbury, Balzer, Childers, & Phelps, 1999; Egan, 2001; Ivey & Ivey, 1998). Numerous re-search studies have indicated that good empathic ability is related to progress in the helping relationship (Carkhuff & Berenson, 1977; Truax & Mitchell, 1971; Neukrug, 1980).

The Carkhuff scale ranges from a low of 1.0 to a high of 5.0 with .5 incre-ments. Any responses below a 3.0 are considered subtractive or nonempathic while responses of 3.0 or higher are considered empathic, with responses over 3.0 called "additive" responses (see Figure 4.1). The original Carkhuff scale in its entirety is reproduced in Table 4.1.

As is obvious in Table 4.1, the Carkhuff scale defines level 1 and level 2 re-sponses as detracting from what the person is saying (e.g., advice giving, not accurately reflecting feeling, not including content), with a level 1 response being way off the mark and a level 2 only slightly off. For instance, suppose a client said, "I can't seem to get along with anybody. People at work seem to avoid me, and my family, well they just are judgmental and yell at me. Life re-

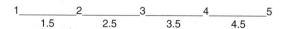

FIGURE 4.1 The Carkhuff Scale

ally sucks." A level 1 response might be, "Well, why don't you do something to make your life better—try harder to get along with people?" (advice giving and being judgmental). A level 2 response might be, "You are having a kind of bad time right now" (does not reflect the intensity of the feeling and is not specific enough about the content). On the other hand, a level 3 response accurately reflects the affect and meaning of what the client has said. Using the same example as above, a level 3 response might be, "Well it sounds like the criticism and yelling at home, as well as people avoiding you at work are making for a really bad time for you right now."

Level 4 and level 5 responses reflect feelings and meaning beyond what the person is saying and adds to the meaning of the person's outward expression. For instance, in the above example a level 4 response might be, "It sounds like you're feeling isolated from everybody at home and at work and pretty down" (expresses new feeling—isolated, which the client didn't outwardly state). Level 5 responses are usually made in long-term therapeutic relationships by expert helpers. They express to the client a deep understanding of the emotions (e.g., intense pain, or joy) he or she feels as well as a recognition of the complexity of the situation.

Usually, in the training of helpers, it is recommended that they attempt to make level 3 response. A large body of evidence suggests that such responses

Table 4.1 Carkhuff's Accurate Empathy Scale

Level 1
The verbal and behavioral expressions of the first person either *do not attend to* or *detract significantly from* the verbal and behavioral expressions of the second person(s) in that they communicate significantly less of the second person's feelings than the second person has communicated himself.

Level 2
While the first person responds to the expressed feelings of the second person(s), he does so in such a way that he *subtracts noticeable affect from the communications* of the second person.

Level 3
The expressions of the first person in response to the expressed feelings of the second person(s) are essentially *interchangeable* with those of the second person in that they express essentially the same affect and meaning.

Level 4
The responses of the first person add noticeably to the expressions of the second person(s) in such a way as to express feelings a level deeper than the second person was able to express himself.

Level 5
The first person's responses add significantly to the feeling and meaning of the expressions of the second person(s) in such a way as to (1) accurately express feeling levels below what the person himself was able to express or (2) in the event of ongoing, deep self-exploration on the second person's part, to be fully with him in his deepest moments.

SOURCE: From *Helping and Human Relations*, Vol. 2, by R. R. Carkhuff, p. 121. Copyright © 1969 Holt, Reinhart & Winston. Reprinted by permission.

can be learned in a relatively short amount of time and are beneficial to clients (Carkhuff, 2000; Neukrug, 1980, 1987). However, for effective empathic responding, it is not only crucial to "be on target" with the feelings and the content but also to reflect these feelings at a moment when the client can absorb the helper's reflections. For instance, you might sense a deep sadness or anger in a client and reflect this back to him or her. However, if the client is not ready to accept these feelings, then timing is off and the response is considered subtractive.

Formula Responses

Often, when beginning helpers first practice empathic responding, it is suggested that they make a "formula response" to client statements. This kind of response generally starts with reflecting the feeling followed by paraphrasing the content. In fact, helpers often call these "reflection of feeling" or "paraphrasing" responses. Look at the example below, and then do Exercise 4.5. In the following example, note how the words "you feel" precede the feelings the client is expressing and the word "because" precedes the content of what the client is saying.

> **Client:** My boyfriend has left me, and I just can't stop crying. I'm so depressed.
>
> **Helper:** You feel *depressed* because *your boyfriend has left you.*

EXERCISE 4.5   Making Empathic Formula Responses

Using a formula response, respond to the scenarios below. In the first few scenarios use the feeling words given to you by the client. However, as the scenarios continue, you will have to imply what the individual is feeling. Try to imply what is obvious; that is, don't try to read to much into the individual's feeling state.

1. Pregnant teenager to human service professional:
   Client: I have to get an abortion. If my parents find out they're going to kill me. If they knew I've been sleeping with John, they'd throw me out for sure. I'm scared.
   HSW: You feel _____ because _____
   _____

2. Individual with a disability to human service professional:
   Client: I'm pissed off. I know they didn't hire me because I'm disabled. I want to know what my legal rights are. Do you know what I can do?
   HSW: You feel _____ because _____
   _____

3. Minority person to human service professional:
   Client: I'm really suspicious. I think I'm getting the shaft with my realtor. I keep telling her I want to move to this one community, and she can't find anything for sale there. I don't believe it!
   HSW: You feel _____ because _____
   _____

4. Teenager to human service professional:
   Client: I'm not worried. My boyfriend doesn't use condoms. Why should he? He's not going to get AIDS—he doesn't sleep around. I'm the only one who sees anyone else!
   HSW: You feel _____ because _____
   _____

5. Abused older person to human service professional:
   Client: I guess I deserve to be hit. I can't remember where I keep anything anymore. Besides, my daughter really loves me.
   HSW: You feel _____ because _____
   _____

6. Accused person to human service professional:
   Client: I didn't do nothing. Those charges are trumped up. They just want to get me because they know I've been in trouble before!
   HSW: You feel _____ because _____
   _____

7. Pro-life person to human service professional:
   Client: I refuse to let any more babies die. I'll do anything to close down those murdering abortion clinics.
   HSW: You feel _____ because _____
   _____

8. Pro-choice person to human service professional:
   Client: I believe a woman has a right to choose what to do with her body, and I'm sick and tired of these pro-lifers interfering with other people's right to choose!
   HSW: You feel _____ because _____
   _____

9. Estranged wife to human service professional:
   Client: My husband wasn't faithful to me so I left him. Now I want him back. I miss him so much. But I can't let him back for what he did to me.
   HSW: You feel _____ because _____
   _____

10. Drug user to human service professional:
   Client: I can stop using. This stuff is not that important to me. If you find me a job, I'll quit!
   HSW: You feel _____ because _____
   _____

Natural Responses

As helpers become more comfortable with formula responses, they can begin to make empathic responses using more natural conversational tones. For instance, in the following example, look at the "natural" response made to the client.

> **Client:** I'm at my wit's end. I'm as depressed as ever. I keep trying to change my life and nothing works. I try communicating better, I change my job, I change my looks. I even take antidepressants, but nothing helps.

> **Helper:** You keeping trying to change your life, but nothing seems to be helping. You're still as down as you've ever been.

Now, using the same scenarios as you used earlier, make natural responses to the situations in Exercise 4.6.

EXERCISE 4.6   Making Empathic Natural Responses

Make a "natural response" to each of the following:

1. Pregnant teenager to human service professional:
   Client: I have to get an abortion. If my parents find out they're going to kill me. If they knew I've been sleeping with John, they'd throw me out for sure. I'm scared.
   HSW: You feel _____ because _____

   _____

2. Disabled person to human service professional:
   Client: I'm pissed off. I know they didn't hire me because I'm disabled. I want to know what my legal rights are. Do you know what I can do?
   HSW: You feel _____ because _____

   _____

3. Minority person to human service professional:
   Client: I'm really suspicious. I think I'm getting the shaft with my Realtor. I keep telling her I want to move to this one community, and she can't find anything for sale there. I don't believe it!
   HSW: You feel _____ because _____

   _____

4. Teenager to human service professional:
   Client: I'm not worried. My boyfriend doesn't use condoms. Why should he? He's not going to get AIDS—he doesn't sleep around. I'm the only one who sees anyone else!
   HSW: You feel _____ because _____

   _____

5. Abused older person to human service professional:
   Client: I guess I deserve to be hit. I can't remember where I keep anything anymore. Besides, my daughter really loves me.
   HSW: You feel _____ because _____

   _____

6. Accused person to human service professional:
   Client: I didn't do nothing. Those charges are trumped up. They just want to get me because they know I've been in trouble before!
   HSW: You feel _____ because _____

   _____

7. Pro-life person to human service professional:
   Client: I refuse to let any more babies die. I'll do anything to close down those murdering abortion clinics.
   HSW: You feel _____ because _____

   _____

8. Pro-choice person to human service professional:
   Client: I believe a woman has a right to choose what to do with her body, and I'm sick and tired of these pro-lifers interfering with other people's right to choose!
   HSW: You feel _____ because _____

   _____

9. Estranged wife to human service professional:
   Client: My husband wasn't faithful to me so I left him. Now I want him back. I miss him so much. But I can't let him back for what he did to me.
   HSW: You feel _____ because _____
   _____

10. Drug user to human service professional:
    Client: I can stop using. This stuff is not that important to me. If you find me a job, I'll quit!
    HSW: You feel _____ because _____
    _____

Advanced Empathy

Sometimes, a helper can make a response that goes deeper than what the client is outwardly stating he or she feels or understands about a situation. When the helper is actually sensing deeper feelings and reflects those, or when, based on the client's statements, the helper can reframe how the client is viewing the situation, the helper has made an advanced empathic response. For example, using the same scenario as earlier, we might find the following response:

> **Client:** I'm at my wit's end. I'm as depressed as ever. I keep trying to change my life and nothing works. I try communicating better, I change my job, I change my looks. I even take antidepressants, but nothing helps.

> **Helper:** Your frustration really shows—you've tried so many different things yet nothing seems to work. I can see your frustration and sadness in your eyes.

In the above example, look at the way the helper reflected the feeling "frustration" that was *not* expressed by the client. As a cautionary note here, helpers should really sense underlying feelings and not reflect "frustration" because they assume that's what the client was feeling. Other times, helpers might use analogy, metaphor, or visual image to bring forth deeper meanings to the client. For instance, in the same situation as above, the helper might say:

> **Helper:** It's kind of like you're rearranging chairs on the *Titanic*. Or,

> **Helper:** When you just told me what you're going through I felt my stomach twist and turn—I imagine this is how you must be feeling.

Generally, it is recommended that beginning helpers try to stick to making formula or natural responses, as making an advanced response is an art that comes with being a seasoned professional. In Exercise 4.7, in small groups, you will have the opportunity to formulate some advanced responses; keep in mind, however, that a good formula response is often as helpful as an advanced response.

Form groups of four or five in your class. Using the same scenarios as earlier, make an advanced empathic response to each of the following:

1. Teenager to human service professional:
   Client: My boyfriend doesn't use condoms. Why should he? He's not going to get AIDS—he doesn't sleep around. I'm the only one who sees anyone else!
   HSW: _____
   _____

2. Abused older person to human service professional:
   Client: I guess I deserve to be hit. I can't remember where I keep anything anymore. Besides, my daughter really loves me.
   HSW: _____
   _____

3. Pregnant teenager to human service professional:
   Client: I have to get an abortion. If my parents find out they're going to kill me. If they knew I've been sleeping with John, they'd throw me out for sure.
   HSW: _____
   _____

4. Disabled person to human service professional:
   Client: I know they didn't hire me because I'm disabled. I want to know what my legal rights are. Do you know what I can do?
   HSW: _____
   _____

5. Accused to human service professional:
   Client: I didn't do nothing. Those charges are trumped up. They just want to get me because they know I've been in trouble before!
   HSW: _____
   _____

6. Minority person to human service professional:
   Client: I think I'm getting the shaft with my Realtor. I keep telling her I want to move to this one community, and she can't find anything for sale there. I don't believe it!
   HSW: _____
   _____

7. Pro-life person to human service professional:
   Client: I refuse to let any more babies die. I'll do anything to close down those murdering abortion clinics.
   HSW: _____
   _____

8. Pro-choice person to human service professional:
   Client: I believe a woman has a right to choose what to do with her body, and I'm sick and tired of these pro-lifers interfering with other people's right to choose!
   HSW: _____
   _____

9. Estranged wife to human service professional:
   Client: My husband wasn't faithful to me, so I left him. Now I want him back. I miss him so much. But I can't let him back for what he did to me.
   HSW: _____
   _____

10. Drug user to human service professional:
    Client: I can stop using. This stuff is not that important to me. If you find me a job, I'll quit!
    HSW: _____
    _____

Practicing Empathic Responses

The more you practice making empathic responses, the better you'll get. Most people don't grow up knowing how to make empathic responses. That is why learning empathy is much like first learning to ride a bicycle—the more we practice, the better we'll get. Exercises 4.8, 4.9, and 4.10 give you an opportunity to practice this very important skill.

EXERCISE 4.8   Practicing Empathic Responding

The following is a scenario of a client named Victoria. For each of the responses make a formula and a natural response. When you have finished, share your responses in small groups and/or in class.

1. Victoria: I wanted to see you today because I felt like my life is falling apart.
   Formula Response: You feel _____ because _____.
   Natural Response:_____
   _____

2. Victoria: Well, since I dropped out of college, I just can't seem to pull things together—not that they were really together when I was in college. But, I can't get a good job, my parents hardly talk with me, and my partner, well, she's always pissed at me.
   Formula Response: You feel _____ because _____.
   Natural Response:_____
   _____

3. Victoria: I've been seriously thinking of just leaving the area and starting all over. Leaving my parents. Leaving Sierra, and leaving it all. Just a fresh start. What do you think?
   Formula Response: You feel _____ because _____.
   Natural Response:_____
   _____

4. Victoria: I guess I'm ambivalent about everything. Maybe I should start college again and try to make amends with Sierra. And, maybe I should sit down and just have a talk with my family. On the other hand . . . I don't know. I just don't know what to do.
   Formula Response: You feel _____ because _____.
   Natural Response:_____
   _____

5. Victoria: Well, I guess I shouldn't be making any rash decisions right at the moment. Perhaps I should just give myself some time and try to sort all of this out in counseling. Yes, I think that's a good idea.
   Formula Response: You feel _____ because _____.
   Natural Response:_____
   _____

6. Victoria: I appreciate your listening to me today. I really feel that I at least have a little bit of a sense of where I'm going. Should I come back next week?
   Formula Response: You feel _____ because _____.
   Natural Response:_____
   _____

EXERCISE 4.9   More Practice with Empathy

The following is a scenario of a client named Jake. For each of the responses make a formula and a natural response. When you have finished, share your responses in small groups and/or in class.

1. Jake: I don't care what you think, I'm not going to go back to that house. My parents just don't understand me. And I won't go back to school either; all they do there is put me in detention all the time. I'm going to fail no matter what I do, so why should I go back!
    Formula Response: You feel _____ because _____.
    Natural Response:_____
    _____

2. Jake: I didn't start that fire, and I didn't steal that car. I get blamed for it all. Nobody ever believes me, and neither will you.
    Formula Response: You feel _____ because _____.
    Natural Response:_____
    _____

3. Jake: I was out cruising with some friends when one of my buddies saw that car. It had the keys in it, and it was running. He just jumped in it and started driving it—I just went along for a ride. What kind of f—king idiot leaves a car like that running anyway? He deserved it to be stolen.
    Formula Response: You feel _____ because _____.
    Natural Response:_____
    _____

4. Jake: So, if you want to get anywhere with me, you'll just leave me alone. No need to do this talking. You won't get anything out of me.
    Formula Response: You feel _____ because _____.
    Natural Response:_____
    _____

5. Jake: What will I get out of this talking anyway? Tell me, what do I get out of it? Like, if you pay me, maybe I'll say something here.
    Formula Response: You feel _____ because _____.
    Natural Response:_____
    _____

6. Jake: The detention center sucks. My parents keep coming to visit me—as if they care. Even my sister comes to see me. It's dark and . . . (begins to sob).
    Formula Response: You feel _____ because _____.
    Natural Response:_____
    _____

7. Jake: Well, I guess I'd like to get out of here. Maybe you could help me get a job or something once I get out. What do you think?
    Formula Response: You feel _____ because _____.
    Natural Response:_____
    _____

EXERCISE 4.10   Empathic Bombardment

Here's a fun exercise to practice empathic responding. Your instructor will sit in the middle of the classroom. Form two circles around him or her. The instructor is the client while the first circle is the "helpers." The second circle is observers who will rate the responses of the helpers. So all of you "observers," make sure you have a pencil and a piece of paper with you. The instructor will role-play a situation and any person in the first circle can respond, but only with an empathic response. The instructor will turn to the "helper" who is responding, and meanwhile, the observers will write down the response and rate it on the Carkhuff scale. After you have done this exercise for a few minutes, observers can share their ratings of the various responses. Then, do another role-play with the observers and helpers switching roles.

Conclusion

Empathy is probably the most important helping skill for the human service professional. It is the skill that works best in building the relationship, is crucial for maintaining a bond with the client, and can help the client understand deeper parts of himself or herself. It is a skill that we are always getting better at as we continue in our careers.

SUMMARY

This chapter examined the important foundational skills of silence and pause time, listening, and empathy. Relative to silence, it is a very powerful skill to use in the helping relationship and allows the client and the helper to review what has been said in an interview. Sometimes, by being silent, clients will want to fill the void and may feel an urgency to talk more fully about a topic. Also, silence is important because when one is not silent, one is not listening. Pause time, which is related to silence, is the amount of time a helper gives between responses. Pause time is cross-cultural in that individuals from different cultures may have varying pause times.

Listening, one of the most important helping skills, is something that does not come easily to many individuals. There are many hindrances to listening, and good listening is facilitative for client growth. Several practical suggestions for listening include talking minimally, concentrating on what is being said, not interrupting, not giving advice, being able to give without expecting to get, accurately hearing content and feelings, communicating effectively that you heard the client, asking for clarification when necessary, and not asking questions.

Empathy is probably the most important skill for the helper. Empathy is the ability to perceive the internal world of the client as if one were the person, "without losing the 'as if' feeling." It has become increasingly important as a helping skill during the twentieth century. Popularized by Carl Rogers, empathy was operationalized by Carkhuff, who developed a five-point scale that delineated different kinds of empathic responses. Those who make a level 3 or higher empathic response are generally helpful to clients; those who make less than a level 3 response may be harmful. A level 3 response was defined as one that accurately reflects the affect and content of what the client is saying. Level 4 reflects feelings and meaning beyond what the client is aware of, and level 5 responses express deep understanding and support. Level 1 or 2 responses are judgmental or off the mark in reflecting affect and meaning.

Making good empathic responses requires learning and practice, beginning with formula responses. These are responses that have a preconceived structure and require the helper to paraphrase content and meaning. Natural responses also reflect content and meaning but do so in a natural and sometimes creative way. Those who are good at empathy are "naturally" empathic and the empathic response is reflected easily to the client.

INFOTRAC COLLEGE EDITION

1. Review how the use of "empathy" and the "Carkhuff Scale" can be used in the "training" of helpers.

2. Research how being empathic can affect one's ability to understand another person.

Commonly Used Skills

INTRODUCTION

The skills presented in this chapter are commonly used by many helpers to assist them in building a strong foundation for the helping relationship. Compared with listening and empathy, in which clients are free to choose what they wish to discuss, the skills in this chapter tend to point them toward certain topics. Thus, the skills of affirmation and encouragement direct clients by reinforcing what they are discussing, and the skills of modeling and self-disclosure encourage clients to focus on specifics topics the helper is modeling or revealing about himself or herself. However, these skills are not nearly as helper-centered as the skills in the next two chapters: questions, advice giving, offering alternatives, and information giving. Nor do these skills have the same potential for creating an authoritarian atmosphere within the helping relationship as do the skills in Chapters 6 and 7. Let's take a look at these skills commonly used by helpers.

AFFIRMATION GIVING AND ENCOURAGEMENT

The need for supporting core self-esteem doesn't end in childhood. Adults still need "unconditional" love from family, friends, life partners, animals, perhaps even an all-forgiving deity. Love that says: "no matter how the world may judge you, I love you for yourself." (Steinem, 1992, p. 66)

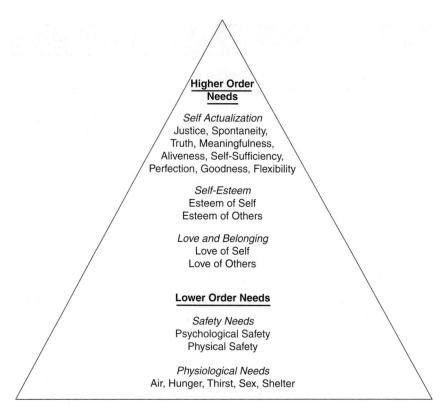

FIGURE 5.1 Maslow's Hierarchy

Many clients who enter a helping relationship are struggling with issues that affect their self-esteem, and this may be the only relationship in which clients may have the opportunity to have their self-esteem lifted. Maslow (1970, 1998) noted that self-esteem is a higher order need—that is, a need of humans that is met only after more basic needs are satisfied. In American culture, for many clients, basic needs have been met; they are struggling with the higher order, more relationship-oriented needs of love and belonging and self-esteem (see Figure 5.1).

The human service professional can actively assist in helping the client feel a stronger sense of love and belonging and in raising the client's self-esteem by affirming the person's self-worth and by encouraging him or her through the helping process. The two most important skills for this are affirmation giving and encouragement.

Affirmation Giving

It is the rare helper who does not affirm his or her clients in some manner. Fleeting statements such as "good job," "I'm happy for you," or strong handshakes, warm hugs, and approving smiles are just a few of the ways in which helpers affirm their clients. Whether called reinforcement or a genuine positive response to the hard work of a client, such relatively minor helper re-

---

EXERCISE 5.1   Giving Affirmations

Part I: The instructor should have the class mingle in an open space. Go up to other students in class and tell them something that you like about them. It could be the way they interact in class, how they dress, how they present themselves, and so forth. See how it feels to offer other persons in class an affirmation.

Part II: The instructor will hand out envelopes and index cards in class. Each of you will write your names on the envelopes and hand them in to the instructor. The instructor will find some place where he or she can post the envelopes and during the week any student can place an affirmation in your envelope. You can either state your name or not. The one rule is that the statement must be positive. Periodically, during the semester, the instructor can process the kinds of affirmations, if any, students are receiving and how they feel about receiving or not receiving affirmations.

---

sponses may greatly affect the client. When helpers are cynical or burned out, or simply have lost their sense of caring for their clients, they are not able to affirm their clients in meaningful ways and may actually be harming them by creating such a negative atmosphere.

Unfortunately, affirmations are not generally handed out freely in many families, and if you did not grow up in an environment that was affirming of you, then you may have difficulty affirming others. However, the good news is that affirmations are easy to make (see Exercise 5.1).

Many clients live in environments where affirmations are rare. Exercise 5.2 lets us determine whether we are receiving affirmations in our lives and can also be used with clients to examine the kinds of affirmations they are, or are not, receiving.

Encouragement

Similar to affirmations, but focused more on helping a client achieve a specific goal, encouragement can also be a vital tool in raising a client's self-esteem. Encouragement includes such helper statements as "I know you can do it" and "Just keep trying." One form of encouragement is for the helper to encourage the client to reach a goal that is determined by the client within the helping relationship. On the other hand, when a helper encourages a client to reach a goal that is *decided on by the helper,* then it is considered advice giving (see Chapter 7 for a discussion of advice giving). Exercise 5.3 gives you practice in using encouragement.

Final Thoughts

Some believe that the use of affirmations and encouragement may begin to form a helping relationship that is based on external validation, which is the validation of self by others as opposed to self-validation (Benjamin, 1987). Helpers must reflect on whether such techniques are assisting clients in the

EXERCISE 5.2 Affirming One Another

On the left side of the paper, write down five things you are good at. Then, on the right side of the paper, write down who, if anyone in your life, has affirmed how good you are at whatever you wrote down. Keep in mind that you might not have always been affirmed by someone on the things that you do. After you have completed writing on the paper, form groups of eight.

Things I'm Good At	People Who Have Affirmed Me
Writing	My Students, Colleagues
Running	My Wife
Discussing Issues	No One
Being a Dad	My Wife, My Daughter, My Mom-in-Law
Being an Administrator	My Dean, My Colleagues

Pick one of the items that you listed. If there was any item that was *not* affirmed by anyone, pick that one. Now sit in the middle of your group, and tell your fellow group members what you do that makes you good at the listed item. Then, have each group member go around and affirm you in that area.

When each member of your group has finished the task, discuss the following issues in your group or in the class as a whole.

1. How did it feel to be affirmed by others?
2. Did you have an easy or difficult time affirming others? Why or why not?
3. Do you find that you are affirmed often in life?
4. Do you think that affirming others, especially clients, would feel genuine?
5. Do you believe that affirmations can really raise a person's self-esteem?
6. Do you think you can increase the numbers of affirmations you give?

EXERCISE 5.3 Encouraging One Another

Get together in dyads and have one student be the helper and the other be the client. The client should discuss a life issue which he or she is having difficulty accomplishing (e.g., losing weight, finding a job, communicating more with a loved one). The helper should encourage the client by saying things like, "I know you can do it," "You have the inner strength to accomplish this," and so forth. After a few minutes, switch roles. After you have completed the exercise, form groups of 8 to 10 students and discuss how it felt to be encouraged by another person.

Remaining in your groups, have one student agree to share his or her life problem with everyone else in class. Have that person sit in the middle of the room, and when appropriate, any class member can encourage the helpee. Class members should only say something if it feels genuine. If time allows, other members of the group can sit in the middle and share their life issues. After the exercise is completed, the "helpee" should discuss how it felt to receive such encouragement.

BOX 5.1   Too Much of a Good Thing?

I once worked with a 16-year-old who had low self-esteem. He had poor social skills and few friends. I often would affirm him and encourage him to try out new behaviors. For instance, I would encourage him to go to the movies, just so he would be getting out of his house. I also would encourage him to call an acquaintance, in an effort to make friends. The work with this young man was slow and tedious, but over time he began to feel a little bit better about himself. I also encouraged him to make positive self-affirmations, which he would practice at home. Thus, he would often say to himself such comments as "I'm worthy and I'm capable." In fact, it began to be a bit of a joke when he would call me "Stuart Smalley," the guy from Saturday Night Live who used to overdo self-affirmations. Finally, when he left counseling he gave me a copy of one of Stuart Smalley's audiotapes to remind me how much I had encouraged him to make those self-affirmations.

---

formation of a higher degree of self-worth or if they may actually be fostering dependency and the continuation of a higher degree of externality. In my own practice, I attempt to find some balance between genuinely affirming a client and my concerns that I might be fostering a dependent relationship.

MODELING

No matter what kind of helping relationship they are in, helpers will act as models for their clients *regardless of whether they want to be or not* (Brammer & MacDonald, 1998). Helpers are constantly modeling for their clients. If they are empathic, then clients may learn how to listen to loved ones more effectively. If they are assertive, then clients may learn how to positively confront someone in their lives. And if they can show a client how to resolve conflict, then clients may learn new ways of dealing with conflict in their lives. By using modeling, helpers can be change agents in two ways, inadvertently or intentionally.

Inadvertent Modeling

The helper who is an inadvertent model does not purposefully set out to change specific client behaviors through the use of modeling. This helper, however, acts as a model through his or her use of helping skills within the relationship. For instance, if a helper is showing empathy toward a client, the client might learn how to exhibit this important skill with others, by experiencing empathy directly from the helper. Or a helper might show good attending behavior, such as eye contact and silence, with a client. The client might learn how to do similar attending to his or her loved ones by having experienced it with the helper. It is common for clients to look up to helpers, even idealize them. Thus, because modeling seems most effective when the model has perceived power, status, competence, and knowledge, helper behaviors may be perceived powerfully by clients (Brammer & MacDonald, 1998). Inadvertent modeling occurs in all helping relationships and should never be underestimated! Exercise 5.4 helps you look at how others have inadvertently modeled for you.

Intentional Modeling

Many helpers use intentional modeling as an important tool in their arsenal of change methods. Intentional modeling offers helpers a number of ways to help clients change targeted behavior (Perry & Furukawa, 1986) including (1) through the deliberate display of specific behaviors on the part of the helper (e.g., expressing empathy, being nonjudgmental, being assertive), (2) through the use of role-playing during the session (e.g., the helper might role-play job interview techniques for the client), and (3) by teaching the client about modeling and encouraging him or her to find models outside the session to emulate (e.g., a person who has a fear of speaking to a large group might choose a speaker he or she admires and view the specifics of how this individual makes a speech).

Intentional modeling involves a two–part process that includes first observing a targeted behavior and then practicing it. Thus, clients need to have appropriate models to mimic *and* need to practice the desired behavior within or outside the session. With intentional modeling, any targeted behaviors the client wishes to acquire need to have a high probability of being adopted. For instance, an individual who has a fear of making speeches would first need to find a model to emulate. After observing this model, a hierarchy could be devised whereby the client would first make a speech to his or her helper, then to some trusting friends, then to a small group, and so forth—perhaps asking for feedback along the way in order to sharpen his or her performance. Using these baby steps helps to assure a high probability of success that the client will adopt the targeted behavior (making speeches).

Intentional modeling is a powerful tool that can be used by helpers to effectively change client behavior. Whereas inadvertent modeling occurs throughout the helping relationship regardless of whether the helper and client realize it, intentional modeling requires a deliberate attempt on the part of the client, in consultation with the helper, to adopt a new behavior. This kind of modeling requires a trusting relationship, should be carefully and deliberately planned, and demands a thorough assessment of the client's needs to assure the appropriate choice of targeted behaviors. Therefore, intentional modeling is generally not used at the beginning of the helping relationship because of the time required to build rapport and establish an accurate assessment of the client and his or her situation. Thus, before doing intentional modeling, helpers

EXERCISE 5.4   Inadvertent Modeling

On the top row of the grid below are individuals whom I have modeled or would like to model. In the space provided in the second row, I have filled in qualities I have taken on from these significant others in my life. In the third row are qualities I have *observed* from others and would like to take on in my life. See how I completed the grid, and in the second grid, fill in the appropriate spaces. If you have additional names you would like to add, create a new grid on a blank piece of paper.

Name of Person You Modeled

	My Father	Roger: My First Therapist	Wife	????
Qualities You Took On from This Person	Integrity: My father was always honest and thoughtful.	Empathy: He was great at exhibiting empathy, and I learned how to be empathic with others by being with him.		
Qualities You Have Viewed and Would Like to Adopt	Patience: He was always soft-spoken and able to avoid making rash decisions.		Slow Eating: My wife eats slowly and savors every bite. I eat too fast and too much.	

Name of Person You Modeled

Qualities You Took On from This Person				
Qualities You Have Viewed and Would Like to Adopt				

EXERCISE 5.5　Intentional Modeling

In the space provided, list the qualities you would like to adopt from Exercise 5.4. Then write out specific ways you could practice the qualities that you identified from your model. In small groups share the qualities and discuss your specific plan for acquiring them. Some groups might want to meet on an ongoing basis to encourage the acquisition of the qualities. How might these qualities work positively for you as a helper?

Qualities You Would Like to Acquire	Mechanism for Acquiring the Qualities Listed
1.	1.
	2.
	3.
2.	1.
	2.
	3.
3.	1.
	2.
	3.
4.	1.
	2.
	3.

---

must establish a strong relationship, perhaps through the use of the essential skills of listening and empathy. Work through Exercise 5.5 for practice in intentional modeling.

HELPER SELF-DISCLOSURE

A former student of mine was in therapy with a psychiatrist who, over time, increasingly began to disclose *his* problems to *her.* One day she heard that he had hanged himself. Following his death she revealed to me that she felt intense guilt that she hadn't saved his life. What a legacy to leave this student! Clearly, the psychiatrist's self-disclosure was unhealthy and unethical. However, despite this unethical self-disclosure on the part of this psychiatrist, under some circumstances, certain amounts of self-disclosure may help a client to open up and may also serve as a model of positive behaviors.

　　Although self-disclosure by helpers can be important and helpful for clients (Kleinke, 1994; Pennebaker, Colder, & Sharp, 1990; Pennebaker & Susman, 1988), when used as a helping skill, it is at best a mixed bag (Don-

---

BOX 5.2   Content Self-Disclosure with a Client

I was working with a client who was sharing some information about her problem with compulsive overeating. As I had struggled with a similar problem, I considered sharing my past difficulties with her, thinking she would feel an increased bond with me and thus trust me more. For about two months I considered sharing my "issue" with her, and then finally noted to her during a session that "I had struggled with compulsive overeating also." She looked at me and without skipping a beat, continued to talk about herself, as if I had never said anything. She wanted to talk about herself, and my issues were irrelevant to her purposes in the helping relationship.

---

ley, Horan, & DeShong, 1990; Doster & Nesbitt, 1979). Kleinke (1994) identifies two types of self disclosure: *content self-disclosure,* in which the helper reveals information about himself or herself; and *process self-disclosure,* in which the helper reveals information about how he or she feels toward the client in the moment.

Content Self-Disclosure

Content self-disclosure, or the helper's revelation of some personal information in an effort to enhance the helping relationship, can have a number of positive results. For instance, such disclosure can show the client that the helper is "real," and can thus create a stronger alliance between the client and the helper. In addition, such disclosure can create deeper intimacy, which ultimately could foster deeper self-disclosing by the client. Finally, self-disclosure of this kind can offer the client new positive behaviors that he or she can model. An example of content self-disclosure might be the following:

> **Helper:** You know, when I went through my divorce, it took me a while to get back on my feet and to enter the social arena again. I wonder if that's what's going on with you?

Notice how in the above example the helper finishes the self-disclosure with a "tentative" question. This is an important technique as it brings the situation back to the client. After all, the helping relationship should be focused on the client, not the helper. In other words, the intent of this kind of self-disclosure is to firm up the helping relationship and enhance the helpee's experience of rapport and trust, not to give the helper and opportunity to talk about himself or herself. However, some clients might feel put off by a helper's temporary focus on self. Others, might feel put off by the helper who shares his or her own troubled times, thinking that helpers should have their act together. Thus, using content self-disclosure should be done with great care after consideration of the client's needs.

Process Self-Disclosure

Similar to the concept of "immediacy," process disclosure involves sharing with the client the helper's moment-to-moment experience of self in relation to the client (George & Cristiani, 1994). Such process comments can have a number of positive effects. For example, they can help clients see the type of impact they have on a helper and ultimately, on others in their lives. Also, they can help clients see how moment-to-moment communication can enhance relationships.

Finally, using process self-disclosure can model a new kind of communication that can be generalized to important relationships in the client's life. Similar to the Rogerian concept of genuineness, process self-disclosure is a mechanism that allows the helper to be real with his or her feelings toward the client. On the other hand, helpers should not confuse such disclosure with the unethical practice of sharing their feelings with a client in an effort to work through their own issues or to achieve catharsis (Rogers, 1957).

Some therapists have cautioned helpers to use care in sharing moment-to-moment feelings with clients. Rogers (1957) pointed out that clients were rapidly changing as they shared deeper parts of themselves, and as they changed, the helper's feelings toward them would likely change also. Instead of sharing moment-to-moment feelings, he suggested sharing persistent feelings, as these are more meaningful to the relationship.

Regardless of the kind of self-disclosure made, its effectiveness is closely related to the way clients view helper self-disclosure and what they expect to gain from it (Derlega, Lovell, & Chaikin, 1976; Neimeyer, Banikiotes, & Winum, 1979; Neimeyer, & Fong, 1983). Therefore, the amount of self-disclosure the helper makes should be directly proportionate to how much the client expects self-disclosure to be a part of the helping process.

When to Use Self-Disclosure

Self-disclosure needs to be done sparingly, at the right time, and only as a means for client growth—not to satisfy the helper's needs (Evans, Hearn, Uhlemann, & Ivey, 1993). I have a general rule that if it feels good to self-disclose, don't. If it feels good, you're probably meeting more of your needs than the needs of your client. Finally, I agree with Kahn (1991):

> I try not to make a foolish fetish out of not talking about myself. If a client, on the way out the door, asks in a friendly and casual way, "Where are you going on your vacation?" I tell where I'm going. If the client were then to probe, however, "Who are you going with? Are you married?" I would likely respond, "Ah . . . maybe we'd better talk about that next time." (p. 138)

Use Exercise 5.6 to practice self-disclosure.

EXERCISE 5.6   Practicing Self-Disclosure

First, students should pair up based on whether they have had one of the following problem situations in their lives.

1. Divorce
2. Getting fired
3. Being "dumped" by a significant other
4. Problem pregnancy
5. Trust issues with friend
6. Financial problems
7. Marital problem
8. Disliking parent(s)

In your dyad, have one person be the helper while the other plays the helpee. The helpee should talk about the chosen situation for 5 to 10 minutes, during which the helper should attempt to make at least one self-disclosing response that relates to the situation. If possible, the response should be given in a manner that would facilitate the client's exploration of self. After you have finished, if time allows, switch roles. In class, address the following questions:

1. Was the helper's self-disclosure helpful to the client?
2. Did the helpee develop a greater alliance with the helper as a result of the self-disclosure?
3. Did the self-disclosure change the focus of the session in any manner?
4. Were there better possible responses than self-disclosure?

SUMMARY

This chapter centered on several skills that are frequently used by helpers: affirmation giving, encouragement, modeling, and self-disclosure. Although commonly used, all these skills can have a positive or negative effect on the helping relationship based on whether they are applied appropriately. Affirming a person can raise his or her self-esteem, and encouraging a client to reach his or her goals can be a useful tool in the helping relationship.

Effective modeling can be done inadvertently or intentionally. Inadvertent modeling occurs when a client picks up a positive behavior of the helper as a by-product of the helping relationship. As an example, a client can learn how to be more empathic because the helper shows empathy within the helping relationship. In intentional modeling, the helper purposely teaches new behaviors that the client can then practice. The most common way to do this is through role-playing.

When helpers use content self-disclosure, they reveal specific facts about themselves to the client in the hope that this information will facilitate a deepening of the helping relationship. Process self-disclosure occurs when helpers and clients share moment-to-moment feelings with one another about the relationship. Some clients are more comfortable with self-disclosure than others, and helpers should try to gauge the client's level of comfort with self-disclosure. Self-disclosure should be used only to enhance client goals and should never be practiced to meet the helper's needs.

INFOTRAC COLLEGE EDITION

1. Research the effects of "self-disclosure" on the helping relationship.

2. Research how "encouragement" has been used in the helping relationship.

3. In addition to the helping relationship, research how "Maslow's hierarchy" has been used as a model in other kinds of relationships.

6

Information Gathering

INTRODUCTION

The skills discussed in this chapter involve ways of gaining information from clients. First introduced is the skill of asking questions. The pros and cons are presented, then distinctions are pointed out among different kinds of questioning techniques, with particular attention to direct questions, closed questions, open questions, and tentative questions. The second part of the chapter explores ways to gather information using a structured interview. Gathering a large array of information from clients when they first enter an agency has become increasingly important. The structured interview can assist the helper in doing this in a timely and thorough fashion.

QUESTIONS

Although asking questions is a skill used frequently with clients, it is often considered questionable by many in terms of effectiveness for client outcomes (Kleinke, 1994; Orlinsky & Howard, 1986). This is partially because asking questions, like the solution-giving skills that will be discussed in Chapter 7, can lead or direct the client, whereas the thrust of the more traditional helping skills is to facilitate a relationship that fosters client self-discovery. In fact, some argue that similar to the solution-giving skills, the use of questions creates a helping relationship that is authoritarian in nature and/or may foster a dependency on the helper as the client begins to rely on the helper to direct the helping relationship (Cormier & Cormier, 1997; Byrne, 1995). Nevertheless, many assert that asking questions can assist clients in quickly identifying and ultimately accomplishing their goals, and that goal attainment will help clients feel better about themselves and deepen the helping relationship. Considering the purpose and the many types of questions in the following sections may help to make this point clearer.

The Purpose of Questions

Why should human service professionals ask questions? Should they ever ask questions? Under what conditions, if any? Can other techniques be used in place of questions? Do questions make a person feel defensive? These are some of the questions about questions.

Although questions are sometimes viewed negatively in training programs (Benjamin, 1987), they can serve a multitude of purposes, which include uncovering historical patterns, revealing underlying issues, gently challenging the client to change, or encouraging the client to deepen his or her self-exploration (Kleinke, 1994). Questions can be asked in many ways, and how they are asked will often determine their effectiveness as a helping skill. Some of the more popular forms include direct questions, closed questions, open questions, and tentative questions.

Direct Questions

A direct question is one the helper asks to get specific information about a topic area. "How many years have you been in the relationship?" or "Can you tell me when you started to feel depressed?" are direct questions because they focus on obtaining targeted information on specific subjects. Which of the following would be direct questions?

1. How do you feel about that?
2. Why do you think that was so important?
3. How many children do you have?
4. Can you tell me more about that?
5. What specifically about the job makes you angry?

From the list above, questions 3 and 5 would be considered direct questions because they focus on content or subject matter—the children, the job situation. Direct questions are helpful when the interviewer needs to obtain factual information quickly from clients, as in an intake interview or when the human service professional is pressured by time constraints to gather information.

Closed Questions

A question that limits the kinds of responses available to the client is a closed question. Closed questions can delimit content or affect.

**EXERCISE 6.1   Contrasting Closed Questions
with Empathic Responses**

Have a student volunteer to talk about a topic of his or her choice. The topic
should involve some kind of life dilemma or difficulty. (Of course, the student
should feel comfortable sharing this information.) Have the class circle around
the student and as he or she talks, and ask him or her closed questions that
delimit content or affect about the presenting issue. Do this for exactly five
minutes, at which point the instructor should shout out "switch." Stop asking
any questions and only make reflective and empathic responses. When you
have finished, discuss the following questions as a group.

1. How did the "helpee" experience the first half of the exercise?
2. How did the "helpee" experience the second half of the exercise?
3. Was it easier for the helpers to ask questions or to make empathic
   responses?
4. How could better questions have been asked?
5. Did questions need to be asked at all?
6. Could better empathic responses have been made?
7. Do you think it would be better to ask a *good* question or to make a *good*
   empathic response?

Closed Questions That Delimit Content The following is a closed question that delimits content: "Did you have one or two jobs last year?" Although
such questions can be helpful if they are on target, they may force the client to
talk about a particular point by pushing the client to choose one of the options given to him or her in the question. What if the client does not want to
discuss how many jobs he or she has held?

Closed Questions That Delimit Affect As an example of an affect-
limiting question, a human service professional might ask a client, "Do you
feel sad or angry? An even more limiting question would be, "What makes
you feel so sad?" These types of questions obviously limit the ability of the
client to respond in a multitude of ways and to reach deep into his or her feeling world (see Exercise 6.1). In general, the closed question is seen as less facilitative than the open question.

Open Questions

In contrast to direct or closed questions, open questions enable the client to
have a wide range of responses. For instance, a client could be asked a question such as, "What are you feeling now?" or "Can you tell me more about
your feelings concerning the end of the relationship?" Open questions can be
very powerful as they allow clients the freedom to respond in a multitude of
ways. This creates an environment in which the client can direct his or her
own session, and thus this type of question is seen as more "client-centered"
than a closed question.

EXERCISE 6.2   Practice with Open Questions

Your instructor should break the class into triads. Within your triad, identify helper, helpee, and observer. The helpee is to choose a topic and the helper should respond by asking only open questions. The observer is there to assist the helper should she or he have difficulty with the task. Also, if the observer believes the helper did not respond with an open question, he or she should stop the interview and the three students should discuss what possible open questions could be asked. Then, resume the exercise. After doing this for 5 to 10 minutes, change roles and have the helpee be the helper, the observer be the helpee, and the helper be the observer. Then, after another 5 to 10 minutes, do the exercise one last time, changing roles again. In class, discuss the relative ease or difficulty of making open questions.

Open questions can also be asked in a manner that allows the client to respond to the content of the interview. Some examples might be, "Can you tell me more about that?" "What do you think that was all about?" "How do you make sense of that?" Exercise 6.2 gives you practice with open questions.

Direct, Open, or Closed Questions—Which to Use? Generally, open questions are more useful than closed or direct questions in facilitating a deeper helping relationship. However, with open questions, the client may not focus on the subject matter about which the helper needs information. For instance, if a helper wants to gather specific family history from the client and asks, "Can you tell me more about your family?" the responses could vary dramatically.

In contrast, the use of a direct or closed question can gather specific information quickly, thus expediting a session. A helper might ask, "Who is in your family and what are their ages?" Or the helper might ask a closed question to understand feelings more quickly. For instance, he or she might ask, "Do you feel good about your family?" The down side to questions like these is that they may direct the session in a manner that is not particularly relevant to what the client wishes to discuss. Thus, the human service professional may sometimes be caught in a dilemma. Does he or she use an open question to facilitate deeper exploration or direct or closed questions in order to gather information quickly?

Tentative Questions

Regardless of the type of question asked, it can be asked in a tentative manner, in which the helper is testing the waters. For instance, rather than saying "Tell me the names of the people in your family and their ages" one could ask, "Would you mind telling me about your family members—their names and ages?" Or rather than asking the closed question "How sad do you feel about your divorce?" a helper could respond with the following tentative question: "I'm wondering if you might be feeling sad right now about your divorce?"

EXERCISE 6.3   Developing Tentative Questions

In class, come up with different beginning phrases that might start a tentative question. For instance, in the previous examples, I began the responses by stating, "I wonder if you . . . ", and with "I would guess that you . . . ". Think of a number of different ways one might begin a tentative question. Write them in the space provided.

1._____

2._____

3._____

4._____

5._____

6._____

These tentative questions lessen the impact of the inquiry and give the helpee an easier opportunity to back out of responding to the question if feeling uncomfortable. Even open questions can be asked tentatively. For instance, rather than saying, "What are you feeling about the divorce?" one could ask, "I would guess that you might have some feelings about the divorce." Sometimes helpers will add a small question at the end such as, "Is that true?"

Sometimes the tentative question is hardly a question at all. It is much more akin to being an empathic response. For instance, in the example above, rather than saying "I would guess that you might have some feelings about the divorce," the helper could ask, "It seems like you're having some feelings about the divorce." Tentative questions tend to "sit well" with clients. They're easier to hear, help the session flow smoothly, help to create a nonjudgmental and open atmosphere, and are generally responded to positively by clients. Use Exercise 6.3 to begin sharpening your skill with tentative questions.

Comparing Direct, Closed, Open, and Tentative Questions

Box 6.1 offers a quick comparison of the different kinds of questions examined thus far in this chapter.

The Use of "Why" Questions

Ever been asked the question, "Why do you feel that way?" Did it make you feel defensive? Because "why" questions tend to make a person feel defensive, it is generally recommended that helpers use other kinds of questions or empathic responses (Benjamin, 1987). If one could honestly answer "why," this would be the most powerful question used in the helping relationship. However, clients use the helping relationship to find the answer to why. If they knew, they wouldn't be in the helper's office. I have found that after I've formed an alliance with a client, I might periodically slip in a "soft" why

BOX 6.1 Comparing Direct, Closed, Open, and Tentative Questions		
TYPE OF QUESTION	**DEFINITION**	**EXAMPLES**
Direct Questions	Questions that focus on specific content in an effort to obtain information quickly.	"If you decide to keep the child, how will you care for it?"
Closed Questions: Delimiting Content	Questions that focus on a particular topic or point of view and force the client to pick between choices given.	"Do you think you will live with your parents or on your own after the child is born?"
Closed Questions: Delimiting Affect	Questions that force the client to pick between feeling choices selected by the helper.	"Did you feel happy or sad when you found out that you were pregnant?"
Open Questions	Questions that allow the client to respond in a myriad of ways.	"How do you feel about being pregnant?"
Tentative Questions	Questions asked in a gentle manner that often allow for a large range of responses from the client.	"Is it that you have a lot of mixed feelings about being pregnant?"

question and say something like, "Why do you think that is?" However, if I use this type of question at all during a session, I use it sparingly.

When to Use Questions

Although questions can be helpful sometimes in uncovering patterns, inducing self-exploration, and challenging the client to change, their careless use can be detrimental. The overuse of questions can set up an atmosphere some consider derogatory in which "the interviewee submits to this humiliating treatment only because he expects you [the helper] to come up with a solution to his problem or because he feels that this is the only way you have of helping him" (Benjamin, 1987, p. 72). Some suggest that questions can lead to an authoritarian atmosphere that fosters dependence on the helper (Cormier & Cormier, 1997; Byrne, 1995). Still others believe that asking a question is not as helpful to clients as making an empathic response (Neukrug, 1999a, 1999b, 2000; Rogers, 1942). This is because a good empathic response is seen as empowering—it allows clients to feel as if they are discovering answers on their own. In fact, an empathic response can often be made in place of asking a question. For instance, suppose a client said the following:

> **Client:** I come in for help from this place, and all I get is a lot of nonsense. No one really wants to help me. No one cares about me, my kids, my family!

A helper could respond with this question:

Helper: Why do you feel that way? Why do you think we don't care?

Although the above responses might be made from a sincere and thoughtful place, they are likely to provoke the client even more, making him or her pretty angry. However, look at the following response:

Helper: It seems like no one here is helpful or cares about you and your family.

Whereas the question is not a bad response, it changes, at least to a minor degree, the direction of the session. Also, questions sometimes can create an authoritarian atmosphere and provoke defensiveness in the client. Empathy, on the other hand, tends to create a nonauthoritarian and liberating atmosphere in which the client feels empowered and heard. Generally, beginning helpers should attempt to make reflective and empathic responses rather than ask questions.

Although much more can be said about the different uses of questions in the interviewing process, remember to be careful whenever you ask questions. Benjamin (1987) suggests the following as a guide:

- Are you aware that you are asking a question?
- Have you weighed carefully the desirability of asking specific questions and challenged their usage?
- Have you examined the types of questions available to you and the types of questions you personally tend to use?
- Have you considered alternatives to asking questions?
- Are you sensitive to the questions the interviewee is asking—is he or she asking them outright?
- Most significantly, will the question you are about to ask inhibit the flow of the interview?

Exercise 6.4 lets you practice your questioning skills.

CONDUCTING A STRUCTURED INTERVIEW

Often when clients first contact an agency they are requested to undergo an initial intake interview to provide background information. The structured interview is one method helpers can use to gather information quickly and accurately. This kind of interview has as its basis a preset format that allows the helper to gather information in a consistent and concise manner. This part of the chapter examines some ways of gathering information using the structured interview format.

EXERCISE 6.4   Asking Effective Questions

For the following questions, decide whether they are direct, closed, open, or tentative. Also, discuss whether some questions could be a combination of these. Finally, offer ways in which you might make a better response than the one given.

Type of Question

Example: Did you feel sad or angry about your   *Closed Question*
              daughter running away?
Better Response: *It sounds like you had some strong*
                     feelings about your daughter's behavior.

Question 1: Did you feel good or bad about the breakup?   _____
Better Response:_____
_____

Question 2: How did you feel about the death of your father?   _____
Better Response:_____
_____

Question 3: How angry were you at your brother for   _____
              not helping you out?
Better Response:_____
_____

Question 4: How many times have you been to the   _____
              unemployment office?
Better Response:_____
_____

Question 5: Is It that you were feeling pretty upset about   _____
              being lied to?
Better Response:_____
_____

Question 6: How often during the day do you cry about   _____
              the breakup?
Better Response:_____
_____

Question 7: Would you like to tell me more about that   _____
              situation?
Better Response:_____
_____

Question 8: Might you have some strong feelings about   _____
              the accident?
Better Response:_____
_____

Question 9: Will it take two or three months to get over   _____
              this?
Better Response:_____
_____

Question 10: Tell me how often you've been in counseling   _____
              and who your counselors were.
Better Response:_____
_____

The Use of Questions in Conducting the Interview

To make the information-gathering process as smooth as possible, ask questions in a manner that is comfortable to the client. Although any type of question already discussed in this chapter can be used, pay attention to how the client is responding. Clients will often respond in a more pleasant fashion to open and tentative questions than to direct and closed questions. However, because direct and closed questions tend to be quicker in obtaining information, they are used more frequently. Be sure to find a balance among these different types of questioning techniques because maintaining a pleasant relationship with your client is as important as gathering information.

In addition to asking questions during the interview, pay attention to your foundational skills. Asking questions of a sensitive nature often touches on many raw areas. Thus, it is crucial that the helper listen attentively and be empathic when painful issues arise. Sometimes you may want to delay gathering information from a client when you feel it is more important to be empathic to a particular issue that has surfaced with the interview questions. Each helper should find a balance among the use of questions, being empathic, and gathering information in a manner that is helpful to the client.

Professional Disclosure Statements and Informed Consent

Generally, when a helper first meets a client, he or she initially makes an introduction and discusses the nature of the interview. Often, this is done by offering clients a *professional disclosure statement,* which is a statement, often in writing, describing the nature of the helping relationship (see American Mental Health Counselors Association, 1987; Corey, Corey, & Callanan, 1998). The professional disclosure statement often includes information about the helping process, the helper's theoretical orientation and credentials, the purpose of the interview, relevant agency rules, limits to confidentiality, legal issues, fees for service, and other important information relative to the helping relationship (Corey, Corey, & Callanan, 1998). The agency itself can develop a professional disclosure statement, but if your place of employment does not have one, develop your own and/or encourage your agency to adopt one (see Exercise 6.5).

After clients have reviewed the professional disclosure statement, the helper should have them give *informed consent* to the interview. Such consent involves verbal or written permission given by the client to participate in the helping interview (see Exercise 6.6).

After giving the client a professional disclosure statement and obtaining informed consent, the helper is ready to gather information. Some information can be gathered by having the client fill out forms; other information requires the helper to ask questions.

EXERCISE 6.5   Developing a Professional Disclosure Statement

Have each student use the outline below to develop his or her own professional disclosure statement. Keep the statement under one page and have a place for your client to sign. After all students have finished, meet in small groups and receive feedback about your professional disclosure statement. Students can then volunteer to read their professional disclosure statements to the whole class.

Explanation of the helping process:

Helper's theoretical orientation:

Credentials held:

Relevant agency rules:

Limits to confidentiality:

Relevant legal issues:

Other:

EXERCISE 6.6   Informed Consent Form

Do either or both of the exercises below:

1. In class, your instructor will choose an agency and discuss the kinds of activities that take place in that agency. Then, as a class, develop an informed consent form for the agency. The instructor will write it on the board.
2. As an alternative, do the same exercise, but in small groups. The class could be broken into small groups based on students' affinity for a particular type of agency. For instance, students who want to work in a rehabilitation agency can form one group, students who want to work in a mental health agency can form a second group, and so forth. After the groups have met, share your informed consent forms with the class.

Gathering the Information

You have handed out your professional disclosure statement and gained informed consent; now you're ready to gather the information. A good method for doing this is to have a preset list you can follow to obtain specific information. Box 6.2 shows several types of information you might want to gather. Of course, the proper use of questions mixed in with your good listening skills will take you far in gathering all the information. When you are ready to begin, Drummond (2000) suggests the following guidelines before and during the interview:

1. Have a clear idea of why the individual is being interviewed. The kinds of questions asked depend on the types of inferences, decisions, or descriptions to be made after the interview. Better information results from specific goals.

BOX 6.2   Outline for Structured Interview

Demographic Information

Name of Client:	Date of Birth:
Address:	Phone (home and work):
E-mail Address:	Current Place of Employment:
Financial Status:	Disability:
Language Spoken:	Race/Ethnicity/Cultural Background:*

*I use this category only if I believe it is relevant to the client's situation. Others use it regularly.

Reason for Referral or Contact
1. Who referred the client to the agency?
2. What is the main reason the client contacted the agency?

Family of Origin Background
1. Relationship with parents or guardians with whom client grew up:
2. Relationship with siblings when growing up:
3. Relationship with significant others when growing up:

Current Family Background
1. Relationship with significant individuals in client's family or extended family (e.g., spouse, significant other, children and stepchildren, others living in current home):
2. Significant events related to family or extended family:

Other Background Information
1. Significant life events:
2. Background to problem:

Cross-Cultural Issues (e.g., client believes he or she is being discriminated against)

Educational and Vocational Background
1. Current employment of client:
2. Describe educational background of client:
3. Describe vocational background of client:
4. Describe educational and vocational background of parents, siblings, and spouse if significant:

Medical/Psychiatric History
1. Health of client:
2. Health-related issues of significant others:
3. History of prior counseling, if any:
4. History of psychiatric admissions, if any:

(Continued)

BOX 6.2   Continued

Substance Abuse History

1. Alcohol:
2. Drug use:
3. Eating disorders:
4. Smoking:

Legal Issues and History

1. Contact with police:
2. Current legal problems, if any:
3. History of any acting out or violent behavior:

Appearance and Mental Status

1. Appearance (grooming, posture, gait, etc.):
2. Hygiene:
3. Nonverbal behavior (e.g., eye contact, rubbing hands together, tics):
4. Speech quality:
5. Orientation: Is the person oriented to time, place, and person? (Does the client know who he or she is, where he or she is, and what time of day it is?):
6. Affect: Describe the client's current feeling state (e.g., happy, sad, anxious, depressed, flat, irritable, hostile, enraged, apathetic, joyful, euphoric):
7. Mood: Describe the client's feeling state of a long period of time (the past year, or even over a lifetime):
8. Cognitive process
   a. Delusions (e.g., Does the person believe he is Jesus Christ?):
   b. Hallucinations (auditory or visual?):
   c. Thought disorder (inability to think in a clear manner, follow conversations, and respond appropriately):
9. Suicidal ideation: Does the client have suicidal thoughts? If yes, ask the following:
   a. In what way has he or she thought of killing himself or herself?
   b. Does the client have a plan developed for killing himself or herself?
   c. Are the tools (e.g., pills, gun) available to the client to follow through on the plan?
   d. If the client has a plan and the tools, how imminent is the suicidal behavior?
10. Homicidal ideation. Does client have homicidal thoughts? If yes, ask the following:
    a. In what way has he or she thought of harming another?
    b. Is there a plan developed for harming another?
    c. Are there tools (e.g., pills, gun) available to the client to follow through on the plan?
    d. If the client has a plan and the tools, how imminent is the event?

EXERCISE 6.7   Practicing Structured Interviews

Each student in the class should find a partner. Have one student be a helper, the other a client. Each helper should first present his or her professional disclosure statement to the client and follow that by giving the client a copy of an informed consent form. Have the client sign the informed consent form. Then, using the your foundational skills (listening and empathy) and your questioning skills, go through the structured interview format listed in Box 6.2. After you have finished gathering information from your client, ask for feedback about how he or she experienced the process. The questions listed below might facilitate the feedback process.

1. Did your client understand your professional disclosure statement?
2. Did your client understand the informed consent form?
3. Did the client feel comfortable during the session?
4. Would the client recommend a greater or lesser use of questions?
5. Did the client feel "heard" during the session?
6. Did the client experience the helper as caring, open, nondogmatic, accepting, and real?
7. Were you able to "build an alliance" with your client through this process?
8. Other feedback?

---

2. Be concerned about the physical setting or environment for the interview. Interviews will go better if the environment is quiet and comfortable. If the room is noisy or has poor lighting, it may detract from the quality of the information gained. Comfortable and private facilities permit the client to relax without the confidentiality and privacy of the interview being threatened.

3. Establish rapport with the interviewee. Good rapport leads the interviewee to be cooperative and motivated.

4. Be alert to the nonverbal as well as verbal behavior of the client. How a person says something may be as important as what is said.

5. Be in charge and keep the goals of the interview in mind. Have the interview schedule readily available but do not suggest answers. Give the client time to answer and do not become impatient during periods of silence. (p. 241)

Exercise 6.7 will help you put together your interviewing skills.

After you have gathered your information, you want to do something with it. Usually, agencies require you to write some type of summary or case report that delineates what you have found, a possible diagnosis, and a treatment plan. In Chapter 8, writing such a report is discussed.

SUMMARY

This chapter discussed important ways to gather information from a client. It examined the use of questions, when questions should be used, if used at all, and the different kinds of questions. There are direct questions, as when the helper is attempting to obtain specific information from a client. There are closed questions that delimit content and closed questions that delimit affect. Such questions limit the kinds of responses the client can make. There are open questions, or questions that allow a wide range of client responses. Regardless of the type of question asked, it can be asked in a tentative manner that tends to "sit" better with the client. In general, the use of questions may lead to a helping relationship that is authoritarian in nature and/or may foster a dependency on the helper as the client is more likely to rely on the helper for directing the helping relationship. Helpers should always consider whether "why" questions should be used at all and when it is best to use any form of a question.

The second section of this chapter examined how to conduct a structured interview as one method of obtaining information from the client. It is important to precede the interview by giving the client a professional disclosure statement and having the client give informed consent to the interview. The use of questions, along with foundational skills, can assist the helper in gathering information from the client.

 INFOTRAC COLLEGE EDITION

1. Find examples of the use of "informed consent" in everyday life.
2. Examine the effect of "interviewing techniques" on your ability to elicit the information being sought.

7

Helper-Centered Skills

INTRODUCTION

This chapter examines a number of helper-centered skills, beginning with the solution-focused skills of offering alternatives, giving information and giving advice. Next, we discuss feedback which can be offered to clients through confrontation and interpretation, and skills for these are described. Last, token economies and other specialized skills are explored. All the helping skills in this chapter are helper-centered; that is, they are focused on the helper leading the session (Benjamin, 1987; Kleinke, 1994).

The down side of using helper-centered skills is that they tend to portray the helper as an expert, encourage externality, and foster dependency. Thus, they are not always effective and should be used only when the helper is pretty confident that they will result in positive client outcomes (Kleinke, 1994; Orlinsky & Howard, 1986). Nevertheless, there are often times when they are appropriate, as when a client is ready to receive feedback and grow from it or when the helper and client have agreed on a specific course of action and the client wants suggestions for moving in that direction. Let's take a brief look at each of these kinds of responses.

SOLUTION-GIVING SKILLS

The helper-centered skills of offering alternatives, information giving, and giving advice can often be used by the helper to assist the client in finding solutions to problems. Helpers are often warned to use these techniques carefully as they have a tendency to lead the client and thus may encourage an overreliance on the helper, thus fostering dependency (Benjamin, 1987; Kleinke, 1994). It is not surprising that some research has shown that these types of skills are not particularly effective (Kleinke, 1994; Orlinsky & Howard, 1986). Even so, at times they are helpful, as when a client wants specific ideas on how to reach his or her goals (e.g., a client who is committed to working on his or her social skills is advised by the helper to join a local community group), or when a client is in crisis and some thoughtful short-term solutions might be helpful (Kleinke,1994).

Offering Alternatives

The first solution-giving skill to be examined, offering alternatives, is when the helper offers realistic choices the client can make in achieving his or her goals. This kind of response suggests to the client that there may be a number of ways to tackle the problem and provides a variety of alternatives from which the client can choose. As compared to information giving and advice giving, offering alternatives has the least potential for harm because it does not presume there is one solution to the problem. It also has the least potential of setting up the helper as the final expert, and to some degree, allows the client to pursue various options while maintaining a sense that he or she is directing the session. Of the three types of solution-giving responses, it is the least judgmental. Work through Exercise 7.1 to learn about offering alternatives.

Information Giving

Information giving, the second type of solution-giving response, offers the client important "objective" information. Because clients often know more than helpers might suspect, the key to making a successful information-giving response is to offer information of which the client is truly unaware. Thus, the information offered should be seen as useful and likely to be used by the client. Because information-giving responses assume that the helper has some valuable information that the client needs, such responses tend to set up the helper as the expert, increasing the potential for the client to become dependent on the relationship. Exercise 7.2 can help you see the pitfalls in information giving.

Offering Advice

The third type of solution-giving response is offering advice: The helper offers his or her expert opinion in hopes that the client will follow up on the suggestions. This kind of response has the potential for developing a depen-

EXERCISE 7.1 Practicing Offering Alternatives

Form triads and in each group have one student be a helper, one a client, and one an observer who will assist the helper, if necessary. The client should talk for a few minutes about a real or made-up problem and the helper is to offer possible alternatives to the client. It is probably best if at first you use your basic listening and empathy skills in an effort to fully understand the problem being presented. Then, after you understand the problem, offer alternatives. The observer can suggest alternatives to the helper if the helper is having difficulty coming up with them. After a few minutes, if time allows, switch roles. If even more time allows, you can switch roles again. After you have finished, discuss in your triad the questions listed below. Students in each triad may want to share their responses with the whole class.

1. Was it easy for the helper to come up with alternatives?
2. Did the client already know the alternatives being offered?
3. Was offering alternatives helpful?
4. Would other techniques have been more helpful than offering alternatives?
5. How did the client react to being offered alternatives?
6. What do you think would have been more helpful to building a foundation to the helping relationship—offering alternatives or another skill?

EXERCISE 7.2 Giving Unnecessary Information

Get into dyads and have one student be the helper and the other the client. The client is to role-play a topic on which he or she is an expert. For instance, if the client worked at Planned Parenthood, he or she might want to role-play a client who is dealing with birth control issues. The helper is to offer information about the topic in an effort to assist the client in finding solutions. For instance, in the present situation the helper might suggest to the client different forms of birth control he or she might try. The client can respond in any way he or she wishes. For example, some clients might respond politely but think to themselves that they are already aware of the information being offered. Other clients might become belligerent, and tell the helper, "I already know about that; you're not helping me." After you've role-played for a few minutes, if time allows, switch roles. After a few minutes, get into small groups to discuss how it felt to be offered alternatives on a topic you already knew thoroughly.

dent relationship as the client could end up relying on the helper for problem solving. In addition, advice giving may mimic control issues from the client's family of origin (e.g., parents giving advice) and is a value–laden response. Some consider advice giving a response that should be avoided (see Benjamin, 1987). However, this response can assist a client in finding solutions quickly. And there are many ways of giving advice. For example, a helper need not act like a tyrant while giving advice (see Exercise 7.3).

> **EXERCISE 7.3   Levels of Offering Advice**
>
> Have one student sit in the middle of three concentric circles. The student in the middle is to role-play a client problem. The innermost circle is to offer advice in a gruff, authoritarian manner. For instance, students in this circle might start responses with statements like, "You should . . . !" or, "It's imperative that you . . . !" The middle circle is to offer advice in a milder form, but still with a dogmatic tone. Some examples of how these students might start responses include "Why don't you . . . " or, "You might want to . . ." The outermost circle is to offer advice in a mild, tentative way while attempting to not be authoritarian. Students in this circle might start their responses with statements like, "I've been wondering if you ever thought about . . . , "or "Have you ever given thought to . . . "
>
> You may want to have a few students take turns sitting in the middle of the circles. After you have done this exercise for 10 or 15 minutes, the students who sat in the middle should share how they experienced each of the circles. Also, individuals in the circles might want to share how they experienced the exercise.

Final Thoughts About Solution-Giving Responses

Although the solution-giving responses of offering alternatives, information giving, and advice giving are similar in the sense that they all move the focus of the session from client to helper, each has a different potential for being possibly destructive to the helping relationship (see Figure 7.1). Clearly, of the three possible leading responses, offering alternatives would be least likely to have a destructive influence. As helpers move toward advice giving, however, they become more value laden in their response mode and more helper-centered, thus potentially more destructive (Doyle, 1997). Whether any of these responses is used within the helping relationship should be based on a careful understanding of the client's needs, and whether an alternative response could be more effective for the client. Meichenbaum (cited in Kleinke, 1994) notes that when the helping relationship is at its optimal, the timing of this kind of response should be such that the client is "one step ahead" of the solution being offered (p. 87). Thus, the client is gaining so much from the helping relationship that he or she comes up with solutions before the helper suggests them.

FEEDBACK

Feedback, the second group of helper-centered skills to be examined in this chapter, can be given to clients in a variety of ways. Two important ways are confrontation and interpretation.

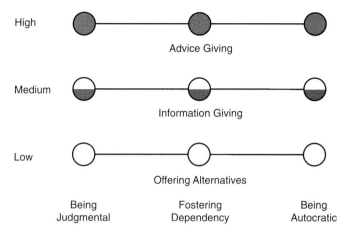

FIGURE 7.1 Potential Level of Destructive Influences of Offering Alternatives, Information Giving, and Advice Giving

Confrontation: Challenge with Support

People generally define confrontation as some type of hostile challenge in an attempt to change another person's perception of reality. However, within the context of the helping relationship, confrontation is generally thought of as a much softer challenge to the client's understanding of the world (Byrne, 1995; Thompson, 1996) and offers the client a method of receiving feedback from the helper. Although one might not realize this if one were to listen to some of the nationally syndicated talk show "therapists," confrontation is *not* (1) yelling at a client, (2) telling a client what to do, (3) acting as if you are the authority figure and have "the answer," (4) laying guilt trips on a client for not accomplishing his or her goals, or (5) acting cynical and treating a person as though he or she is not worthwhile.

   To be effective, confrontation within the helping relationship first involves the building of a trusting and caring relationship. The use of good listening skills and empathy is generally considered to be the most effective way of developing such a relationship. The building of such a relationship is then followed by gentle prodding that carefully pushes the client toward change. This mild confrontation lessens the likelihood that any psychological harm will occur to the client (Egan, 2001; Kleinke, 1994; Young, 1992). This process of support followed by a challenge offers the best potential to change the client's perception of reality (Neukrug, 2000).

   Sometimes, I have found that clients "hook" me, and I start to argue with them about how to live life. This kind of confrontation is rarely, if ever, helpful to the client and is almost always a result of some unfinished business of the helper. Effective helpers have the ability to distance themselves from these emotional entanglements and are able to build effective relationships that offer the potential to change the client's understanding of the world.

Highlighting Discrepancies When Confronting Clients

Confrontation in the helping relationship can assist the client in seeing discrepancies among his or her words, feelings, and/or behaviors. Hackney and Cormier (2000) and Neukrug (1999a) have highlighted discrepancies between a client's (1) *values* and *behavior,* (2) *feelings* and *behavior,* (3) *idealized self* and *real self,* (4) *expressed feelings* and *underlying feelings* of which the client is unaware. Let's briefly examine each of these potential client discrepancies followed by ways of confronting them.

Discrepancy Between a Client's Values and Behavior   When a client expresses a certain value and then his or her actions do not match that expressed value, there is an incongruency within the client. For instance, suppose a client has been an anti-abortion advocate, and then tells you one day that her 15-year-old daughter is pregnant and she is "making her" get an abortion. Pointing out the discrepancy to the client might assist her in either reformulating her values or in changing her behavior (making the daughter get an abortion). However, how the incongruency is presented to the client is important. For instance, one helper might say:

"You told me you were against abortion. Why are you doing this?"

Such a confrontation might make a client defensive. However, another helper could say:

"That's interesting. I was under the impression that you were against abortion. Help me understand."

Discrepancy Between a Client's Feelings and Behaviors   Sometimes a client might assert certain feelings and then act in a manner that seems to indicate otherwise. For instance, suppose a spouse tells a helper that he loves his wife, and then goes on to note how often he beats her and cheats on her. As with pointing out discrepancies with values and behaviors, the helper can further client self-realization by noting such inconsistency.

Discrepancy Between Idealized Self and Real Self   Some clients might idealize the ways in which they would like to act and then find excuses as to why they do not actually act in that manner. For instance, a client might state that he wants to be more real in relationships and then state that he can't be honest with people because if he was really honest, others would not like him. Or a client might state, "I want to communicate effectively with others" but then find reasons for not acting in that manner: "If only I had more time to work on my communication problems."

Discrepancy Between Expressed Feelings and Underlying Feelings A fourth type of discrepancy is between a client's verbal expression of feelings and the underlying feelings a client won't admit or is not currently aware of—for instance, a client who states she is not feeling anxiety related to her marriage and yet seems to be holding back tears. The helper notes this discrepancy and she begins to sob.

Ways of Confronting Client Discrepancies

A helper can confront a client in several ways that gently prod him or her to examine behaviors, thoughts, and feelings. Prior to any confrontation, the helper must first use his or her basic skills to build a strong helping relationship. After this foundation is formed, the helper can use any of the following ways to point out discrepancies:

1. *You/But Statements.* When confronting a discrepancy in this manner, the helper verbally identifies the incongruence through the use of a "you said/but" statement (Hackney & Cormier, 2000). This will make the client face his or her discrepancy and alone may be sufficient to convince the client to change. For instance, to a client who says he believes in honesty but is having an affair, the helper might state:

   Helper: You say that you believe in honesty, but you seem to be hiding a serious matter from your wife.

2. *Asking the Client to Justify the Discrepancy.* Another way of pointing out a discrepancy is to request gently that the client justify the contradiction by having the client discuss the inconsistency of it. For example, in the above example the helper might say:

   Helper: Help me understand how on the one hand you say you are honest, and on the other hand you are hiding an affair from your wife?

3. *Reframing.* This way of highlighting the discrepancy challenges the client to view his or her situation differently by offering an alternative reality.

   Helper: Even though honesty is important to you, sometimes other values override your desire to be honest. So, in this case your value of protecting yourself and your wife from the pain of the affair may be more important than your value of being honest.

4. *Using Satire.* A fourth way a helper could point out a discrepancy is through the use of satire. Highlighting the contradiction in this way is more confrontational than the other techniques and should be done carefully, if at all. The absurdity of the discrepancy is confronted. For instance, in the above example, you might say:

   Helper: Well, I guess it's okay in this instance to be dishonest, after all, you're saving your wife from those painful feelings. Aren't you???

Confronting Sally

Sally made almost $70,000 a year and was in a verbally abusive relationship. Even though she had no major bills, she insisted that she could not leave the relationship and live on a "meager" $70,000 a year. Clearly, her verbal statement that she could not leave the relationship did not match the reality that almost anyone could live on this amount (certainly, most of us would be happy to do so). After building a relationship using empathy, I gently challenged this perception. I did this by using many of the techniques above. Using "You/But" statements, I pointed out the obvious discrepancy between her salary and her ability to live on her own. Also, I gently asked her to justify to me how she could feel this way. This assisted her to see that her logic did not hold up. Using higher-level empathy I reflected back a deeper issue that I experienced her saying—that she felt as if she was a failure in the relationship and was scared to be alone (she was a recovering alcoholic and was concerned she would start drinking again if alone). I encouraged her to work on communication issues with her lover. At the same time I assisted her in reframing her situation so that she could believe that she could live on her own—if she eventually chose to do this. I did not use satire with her, as I felt it would be too disturbing for her. The result for this client was that she became a more assertive woman who improved her communication with her lover and could realistically see her choices about staying in the relationship or finding a place on her own.

---

5. *Higher-Level Empathy.* The final way of challenging a client's discrepancy is through the use of higher-level empathic responses. By reflecting to the client feelings and conflicts that are deep and out of his or her awareness, this kind of response challenges the client to expose deeper parts of himself or herself. For instance, in the above example:

Helper: You must be feeling quite conflicted. On the one hand you say you believe in honesty; on the other hand, you are hiding an affair. I guess I sense there is more to this story for you.

Use Exercise 7.4 to begin working with client discrepancies.

Interpretation

A client offers details about his significant other. Later he shares details about his relationship with his parents. The helper hears similar themes and feelings running through these relationships and reveals the analysis to the client. The client shakes his head in agreement. Is this interpretation or is this empathy? Although some may consider this interpretation (Benjamin, 1987; Cormier & Cormier, 1997), this could very well be a high-level empathic response (Carkhuff Scale, above 3.0) for a number of reasons. First, it is a result of deep

---

EXERCISE 7.4 Responding to Discrepancies

Using the discrepancy categories discussed earlier in the chapter [(1) *values* and *behavior,* (2) *feelings* and *behavior,* (3) *idealized* and *real self,* (4) *expressed* and *underlying feelings*], generate a list of client scenarios. The instructor should summarize the scenarios on the board.

Next, have students form small groups, with each group representing one of the five ways to confront discrepancies (see below). In your small groups, come up with responses to the client using the confrontational technique assigned to your group and write them in the space provided. When you have finished in your groups, pick a spokesperson and have that person share the responses. If time allows, have each group take one or more of the other techniques and make additional responses to those techniques. Share them in class.

Group 1: You/But Statements:

Group 2: Asking the Client to Justify the Discrepancy:

Group 3: Reframing:

Group 4: Using Satire:

Group 5: Higher-Level Empathy:

---

listening and concentration by the helper. Second, it is based on a deep understanding of the *client's framework of reality.* Third, the helper has reflected back an understanding of the client's predicament without adding material that was not stated by the client and without jumping to conclusions or making assumptions. And finally, the client agrees with the helper's assessment. The helper is "on target" with the response. This type of response is profound, reaches deep inside the client's soul, and speaks to the imaginary line between facilitating and leading a client (Benjamin, 1987).

On the other hand, contrast the above helper response with the helper who states, "I believe your relationship with your lover is the result of deep-seated anger stemming from your unresolved oedipal complex." This kind of interpretation is the analysis of a client from the perspective of the helper and is based on a preset model of counseling and psychotherapy that makes assumptions about how a person would react under certain circumstances.

Psychoanalysis uses interpretation as a major therapeutic intervention. For instance, psychoanalysts believe that dreams hold symbols to unresolved conflicts from our psychosexual development and can provide the client with understanding into his or her development (Brill, 1985). A dream about a goat being a person's pet in an immaculately clean apartment could represent an underlying need to rebel against a repressive upbringing, the goat representing the archetypal oppositional animal. Similarly, some cognitive therapists assume that individuals with specific diagnoses would be expected to have certain kinds of underlying cognitive structures (ways of thinking) that can be interpreted to the client (Lynn & Garske, 1990). For example, it would be assumed that a person with an anxiety disorder has an underlying belief that the world is a fearful and dangerous place.

Whether one is psychodynamically oriented, cognitively oriented, or relying on some other theoretical approach, the timing of the interpretation is crucial, with the result—if all goes well—being a deeper understanding of why the client responds the way he or she does, an understanding that should lead to client change.

Although interpretations may assist the client in making giant leaps within the therapeutic context, there are risks involved in using this technique. For instance, interpretation sets the helper up as the "expert" and lessens the realness of the relationship (Kleinke, 1994). In addition, it lessens the here-and-now quality of the therapeutic relationship while increasing the amount of intellectualizing that occurs during the session as both the helper and client discuss the interpretive material (Safran & Segal, 1996). Finally, research does not show strong evidence that interpretation is related to successful client outcomes (Orlinsky & Howard, 1986). It is for these reasons that Carl Rogers and others (e.g., Benjamin, 1987; Kahn, 1991) vehemently opposed the use of interpretation.

> To me, an interpretation as to the *cause* of individual behavior can never be anything but a high-level guess. The only way it can carry weight is when an authority puts his experience behind it. But I do not want to get involved in this kind of authoritativeness. "I think its because you feel inadequate as a man that you engage in this blustering behavior," is not the kind of statement I would ever make. (Rogers, 1970, pp. 57–58)

Whether you believe in the use of interpretation most likely depends on your view of human nature. If you align yourself with a model of counseling that makes assumptions about human behavior external to the client's understanding of reality, then interpretation of client material will become an important tool for you. On the other hand, if you assume that client growth is based on clients' obtaining a fuller understanding of themselves from their own view of reality, than interpretation is likely to be a useless tool for you in the helping process. Finally, if you do believe interpretation can be a valuable tool in the helper's repertoire, then clearly it should be used only after a trusting relationship has been established and with a sound knowledge of the theoretical approach you follow.

EXERCISE 7.5   Being Sigmund Freud

Have a student volunteer to act as if she or he is a Freudian analyst. As such an analyst, feel free to make ongoing interpretations to a role-playing client. You may want to use the list below to help guide you in making interpretations.

1. If the client talks about a dream, interpret aspects of the dream to mean something significant about the client's life.
2. Explain current relationship issues as being caused by the client's relationship with his or her parents.
3. Discuss how current relationship issues relate back to the client's first five years of life, particularly how the client was parented.
4. Interpret client defensiveness and resistance as a mechanism for the client to avoid talking about deeper issues.
5. Interpret most client actions as the client's unconscious means of getting his or her needs met.
6. If the helper is familiar with Freudian theory, use other interpretive techniques in addition to the those listed in items 1–5.

After the role-play is finished, discuss with the client and the class the following questions.

1. What is the likelihood that the interpretations were "on target"?
2. How did the client feel when the helper made the interpretations?
3. How can such interpretations be helpful? Harmful?
4. How thoroughly does one need to understand a specific theoretical model to make good interpretations?

When to Use and Not Use Interpretation

Because interpretation requires in-depth knowledge of an associated therapeutic approach, helpers should use this technique only if they are thoroughly trained in a specific approach that relies on interpretation (e.g., psychoanalysis). Most human service professionals do not have the type of training needed to use interpretation wisely. In fact, beginning helpers sometimes use interpretation capriciously, which can be seriously detrimental to a client. Do Exercise 7.5 to see how interpretation can be used in a negative manner.

Unlike many of the skills discussed in this text, interpretation is one that I recommend you do not use in your repertoire of helping behaviors—for a number of reasons. First, interpretation has not been shown to be significant in improving client outcomes. Second, to use interpretation effectively, helpers must have a thorough knowledge of the theoretical model on which the interpretation is based. Most human service professionals do not have that level of training. Finally, too many human service professionals use interpretation in a haphazard manner, making up their own interpretations as they go. Now that you know what interpretation is and how it can be used incorrectly, examine how you work with your clients and try to *not* use this technique (see Exercise 7.6). If you use the other techniques discussed in this text, you will be well on your way to helping clients.

EXERCISE 7.6   Are You Using Interpretation?

To examine whether you tend to offer interpretations, break up into groups of four and have one student be the helper, have one be the client, and have two observe. The client is to discuss a real or made-up problem situation. The observers are to write down each helper response that appears to be either not related to what the client is saying or to be interpretive leaps that tend to explain client behavior through some external model. The observers might also want to use the list below as a guideline to determine whether the helper is making interpretive responses. When you have finished, discuss the helper responses in small groups. If time allows, switch roles.

1. Keep track of how many times the helper asks "Why" questions. Why questions are often attempts to try to relate client responses to imagined events.
2. Are responses not directly related to what the client is discussing?
3. Is the helper trying to connect the client's discussion to some event the client has not mentioned?
4. Does the client seem not to understand helper responses?
5. Does the helper seem convinced that the client's problems lie elsewhere, such as in issues the client is not discussing?

SPECIALIZED SKILLS

Many other helper-centered skills can facilitate client learning and personal growth. The use of token economies is such a skill. Others would require training beyond the traditional undergraduate human services program. All the skills discussed here are helper-centered—that is, they allow the helper to direct the client.

Token Economies

The behavioral technique of establishing a token economy has been successfully used with different client populations, particularly the mentally retarded. This technique is based on operant conditioning, a type of learning theory, and uses reinforcement contingencies to change client behaviors. The token is considered a secondary reinforcer and can become quite powerful in changing behaviors because it is associated with a desired object for which the token is being exchanged.

Typically, with this technique, a client is given a token for specific targeted behaviors that he or she is asked to exhibit. For example, a person might receive a token for successfully getting dressed in the morning, for exhibiting "appropriate" personal traits, for bathing himself or herself, and so forth. At the end of a specified amount of time, such as a day or a week, the individual can trade in his or her tokens for money or some other reinforcer such as candy or items in a gift shop.

> ### James's Day at the Group Home: A Typical Scenario of a Token Economy
>
> James wakes up in the morning and after successfully dressing himself is given a token. He has a special pouch where he keeps his tokens and he generally beams proudly upon receiving one. After dressing, he eats breakfast with the other members of the group home and then completes his task for the day, which may include doing the dishes, taking out the garbage, or clearing the table. When he completes each task, he is given another token. James's day is very structured and includes specific activities, depending on the day of the week. As this is a Monday, James attends reading group in the morning, when volunteers read stories to the members of the group home. Sometimes, some of the group members read stories to one another.
>
> After lunch, James and the other group members will go on their weekly walk picking up trash along the side of the road near their group home. They have a special sign on the road that notes that this road is kept clean by their group home. They are all very proud of this sign. During the day James can continue to receive tokens for assisting with the meals and for exhibiting good (appropriate) behavior. Tokens are never taken away from group members, but all of the group members know that if they do not behave in the "right way," they will not receive a token. James usually receives about 8 tokens a day, and every Saturday he can exchange the tokens for a gift. The group home has a small area of a room with a number of gifts the members can view. They range from things like stuffed animals to books to calculators.

Although token economies have been quite successful when applied to group homes for the mentally retarded, they can also be highly motivating for other populations, including children, the mentally ill, and even college students. See how you might be able to apply the token economy in your class (Exercise 7.7).

Brief Treatment

One recent major focus has been to offer clients treatment in a short amount of time (Preston, Varzos, & Liebert, 2000). Pressure to offer brief treatment is coming from many places, such as health care organizations that want helpers to limit sessions, schools that view counseling as short term, and agencies that often have a limited number of helpers to work with a large number of clients. Generally, the helper-centered skills discussed in this chapter have become popular because they tend to move the helping relationships along quickly. Such helper-centered skills place the helper in the role of decision maker who must determine (1) the goals of treatment, (2) the approach to take with the client, and (3) how to reach client goals in a short amount of time. Brief treatment approaches, including the use of the helper-centered skills in this chapter, are not without their critics as they are believed by some to create an authoritarian atmosphere in the helping relationship, to lend themselves to

---

EXERCISE 7.7   Applying the Token Economy to Your Classroom

This exercise can be accomplished in groups of five to eight students, or in the class as a whole. The instructor should decide whether the token economy will be used for one class, a number of classes, or the rest of the term. The instructor should also have acquired a number of tokens that he or she will disburse when appropriate behavior is exhibited (the dollar store usually works just fine). Whether it is the whole class or small groups, the following steps must be completed.

1. As a class, discuss how long the experience will take place (a class, two classes, the rest of the term).
2. Decide what behaviors will be reinforced (e.g., you could reinforce coming to class on time, not talking in class, answering a question correctly, being kind to others, participation, and so forth).
3. Clearly define the behaviors that are being reinforced.
4. Decide what types of prizes are to be obtained for the behaviors being reinforced and decide how many tokens it takes to obtain a prize.
5. Make sure everyone has the opportunity to obtain a prize if he or she exhibits the correct behaviors.

---

dependent client-helper relationships, to be lightweight, and to offer short-term solutions to long-term problems (Wylie, 1995). Clearly, the human service professional of today must balance the need to use brief-treatment, helper-centered skills that will solve problems in the short term with the need for long-term solutions to in-depth client problems (Dryden & Feltham, 1992). Often, this is not an easy balance to achieve.

Other Specialized Skills

There are many other kinds of skills that a helper may find useful. From neural linguistic programming, to multimodal therapy, to cognitive techniques, to Jungian and other neo-Freudian techniques, the list is remarkably long. However, learning these very specialized skills is not the focus of a book such as this. At some point, when you advance in your training, you might want to examine some of these more elaborate, in-depth skills and add them to the repertoire of the basic skills that you have learned in this text.

SUMMARY

This chapter examined helper-centered skills including three important solution-giving skills: offering alternatives, information giving, and offering advice. Offering alternatives provides the client with multiple alternatives to choose from, information giving provides valuable information of which the client is not aware, and advice giving offers the client specific solutions to problems. All three have the potential for being destructive to the helping relationship in that they are all value laden, can foster a dependent relationship, and can set up the helper to be autocratic. Advice giving has the most potential for being destructive, offering alternatives has the least; but these responses can be softened, thus increasing their possible effectiveness.

Feedback, another helper-centered skill, was shown to be offered through confrontation and interpretation. Confronting a client must be done in a supportive counseling relationship. Among the discrepancies clients might present to the helper, which the helper may confront, are discrepancies among the client's values and behavior, feelings and behavior, idealized self and real self, and expressed feelings and underlying feelings. Five ways of confronting such discrepancies were offered.

Interpretation, the second method of offering feedback, should generally be avoided by beginning human service professionals. Although an important technique used by some advanced mental health practitioners, interpretation is often used unwisely and capriciously by beginning helpers. Interpretation was defined, some of the pitfalls of using it were discussed, and ways were offered to determine whether you are making inappropriate interpretive responses.

Some specialized skills examined were the use of token economies and the whole area of brief treatment. In addition, it was noted that many other specialized skills could be learned in advanced training.

Helper-centered skills can be effective in helping clients reach specific goals; however, they can also encourage externality, foster dependency, and set up the helper as an expert who might solve short-term problems at the expense of long-term solutions.

SPECIAL INTEGRATION OF SKILLS EXERCISE

1. In Appendix C you will find a listing of the skills from Chapters 4 through 7 and how they are associated with each stage of the helping relationship. Examine the summary and then complete the exercises related to each stage of the helping relationship.

 ## INFOTRAC COLLEGE EDITION

1. Research any specialized skill you want to learn more about.
2. Examine the use of "interpretation" in the helping relationship.
3. Review the efficacy of "token economies" with varying client populations.

Treatment Issues

The last section of the book examines treatment issues, many of which are unique to the human service professional. Chapter 8 describes nine important case management issues covering the entire spectrum of treatment from diagnosis to follow-up. The last two chapters of the section explore the importance of cross-cultural understanding to the effective helper, and review ethical and professional issues relevant to the human service professional.

8

Case Management

INTRODUCTION

This chapter examines the broad range of activities known as case management, which has been viewed as the overall process involved in maintaining the optimal functioning of clients (Sullivan, Wolk, & Hartman, 1992; Woodside & McClam, 1998). Case management involves such things as (1) treatment planning: assessing needs and developing goals (2) diagnosis, (3) monitoring the use of psychotropic drugs, (4) case report writing, (5) managing and documenting client contact hours, (6) monitoring, evaluating, and documenting progress toward client goals, (7) making referrals, (8) follow-up, and (9) time management. With an increased emphasis on accountability in the mental health professions, these issues have become increasingly important. Let's take a look at each of the activities that make up the broad area called case management.

TREATMENT PLANNING

The two major areas of treatment planning—assessment of client needs and formation of client goals—are intimately related. A poor assessment of client needs will lead to inadequate development of client goals.

Assessing Client Needs

Accuracy in assessment of client needs is crucial if appropriate goals are to be set. As helpers develop more ways to assess clients, their ability to set accurate goals will increase (Drum, 1992; Goldman, 1992; Hohenshil, 1993). Ideally, assessment involves a range of information-gathering activities that can include (1) the clinical interview, (2) testing, (3) observation, (4) client self-assessment, (5) assessment of the client by others, and (6) review of past records (Harrington, 1995). A continuous and ongoing process (Vacc, 1982), assessment tends to move from being helper-centered, in the sense that the helper provides the tools to assist clients in their own self-assessment process, to being client-centered, whereby clients have learned how to assess themselves. Capable self-assessment often means that the helping relationship is near its end as the seeds have been planted for clients to continue with an ongoing and deepening reflection process throughout their lives. Six areas of assessment are identified for study here.

The Clinical Interview Probably the most important area of assessment, the clinical interview allows the helper to gather basic information directly from the client. Often, this interview takes place during the initial contact with the agency and is called an "intake interview." This interview must be completed in a manner that will allow the client to be open and honest with the helper so that understanding of client issues is clear and comprehensive. Of course, the helping skills and techniques discussed throughout this text are the basis for the clinical interview.

Testing An important aspect of the assessment process, testing can be done in formal and/or in informal ways. Formal testing involves the use of standardized, well-designed tests whereas informal assessment can involve such things as observation, helper-made ratings scales, or behavioral checklists. In either case, testing is generally talked about as being in two realms: the cognitive and the affective. Cognitive testing measures the client's ability in the areas of achievement, what the client has learned; and aptitude measures what the client is capable of learning. Affective testing, often called personality assessment, assesses the client's temperament and likes and dislikes. In some cases personality assessment can garner information from clients that they are not aware of or that they are purposely hiding (e.g., a client may reveal signs that he or she is a child molester through certain kinds of personality assessment). Although the human service professional is not generally trained to administer advanced types of tests, he or she should still use available assessment results, such as prior testing records.

Observation Sometimes considered a subclass of testing (see Drummond, 2000), observation allows the helper to view client behaviors directly. Because the isolation of the office can at times blur the true nature of a client's behavior, observation of the client in his or her natural environment can be eye opening. For instance, if the helper is working with a child, observing him or her at school or at home can increase the helper's understanding of the child.

Even with adults, if the helper can observe the client "in vivo" he or she will have a better sense of the client.

Client Self–Assessment   Often, the best person to assess the client is the client. This can be accomplished in a number of ways including journaling, keeping a diary, keeping a sleep journal, writing a self-assessment of abilities, writing a self-assessment of strengths and weaknesses, completing a lifeline, and so forth (complete Exercise 8.1).

EXERCISE 8.1   Completing a Lifeline

Pair up with a student and develop a lifeline like mine below. Start with your birth, with the midpoint being satisfaction, the upper point being ecstasy, and the lower point being deep depression. After you have completed your lifeline, discuss your "ups and downs" with your partner. Each student should feel free not to discuss a particular event. In that case, just say to your partner, "I'll pass on that."

After you have completed the lifeline, do the second lifeline below. In this case, draw a straight line from your birth to your current age. Write your current age at the end of that line and then draw a staggered line from your current age to the age which you think you might die. Then, discuss with your partner how satisfied you are with your life to date and what you want to do to make your life complete before you die.

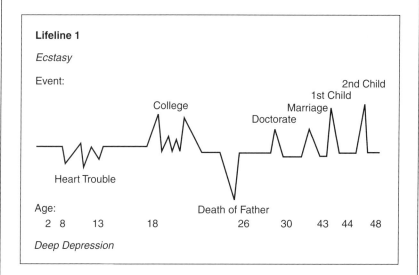

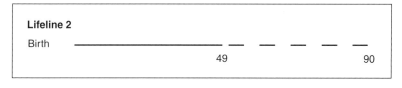

Assessment of Client by Others Generally, there are many people in a client's life who know the client fairly well. Sometimes these people will know aspects of the client better than the client, thus professionals may discuss clients with people who have extensive knowledge of them. For instance, it is typical for parents and teachers to be consulted when the helper is working with a student, and when working with adults, it is not unusual to include spouses, significant others, and family members in the assessment process.

Review of Client Records Today, there is a staggering amount of information on record about each of us. It would be a great error not to attempt to gather some of this information when doing a thorough assessment. It is often suggested that helpers request records from agencies, schools, or other places (e.g., income statements, divorce papers). Sometimes, if a professional does not want to be overly influenced by the opinion of others, he or she will form preliminary opinions prior to obtaining records. Then, after obtaining the records, the professional can see whether they validate his or her judgment.

Developing Client Goals

The actual development of client goals should be a relatively easy process if the helper has completed a thorough assessment of the client. In developing goals, the following should be considered:

1. Goal development should be a natural outgrowth of the assessment process.
2. Goal development should be collaborative. Goals should not be "given" to the client.
3. Goals need to be attainable. If too lofty, the client will feel like a failure if they are not met. If too simple, they are less likely to help the client feel successful.
4. Monitor progress toward goal attainment. If the helper never checks to see whether goals have been accomplished, the client might question the helper's ability or might feel as if the helper does not care for him or her. Lack of goal attainment needs to be reviewed to determine whether goals need to be changed.
5. Goals can be changed. If a client is not reaching his or her goals, discuss why. Were they too difficult or too easy? Were they the wrong goals? Were they not attempted due to lack of time or motivation? After determining why they were not reached, rework the goals and try again!
6. Reinforce the attainment of goals. Clients work hard to reach their goals and it is important that they are affirmed for their success. Clients can be affirmed verbally, through small awards (e.g., a certificate), and in other ways.
7. Develop new goals as former goals are reached. As clients reach their goals, determine whether they are ready to work on new ones.

EXERCISE 8.2   Assessing Needs and Developing Goals

Part I: Spend 10 to 20 minutes interviewing another student who is role-playing a client or discussing a real situation. While interviewing your client, assess the client's needs. When the interview is near completion, write down the client's needs as you view them. After you have finished, obtain feedback from your client as to the accuracy of your assessment.

Part II: Spend a minimum of 10 minutes developing your client goals. The goals should be an outgrowth of your client's needs that were formulated in Part I. Make sure that the goal-setting process is collaborative and that the client is comfortable with the ones developed.

---

8. Know when to stop. Although it is important to keep clients moving forward, also know when to encourage a client to stop. Sometimes a client has simply finished!

Work through Exercise 8.2 to help you with client assessment and goal development.

DIAGNOSIS

A diagnosis is a natural outgrowth of the assessment process and can occur in many ways. For instance, helpers can make an informal diagnosis to be used in goal setting, a rehabilitation diagnosis for physical problems, a vocational diagnosis for career planning, a medical diagnosis, and a mental health diagnosis, such as those made from the *Diagnostic and Statistical Manual of Mental Disorders* Fourth Edition Text Revision (DSM-IV-TR) (American Psychiatric Association, 2000). Because the DSM-IV-TR diagnosis has become an increasingly important part of the assessment process, it warrants a more in-depth discussion.

Why Use *DSM-IV-TR?*

With evidence that a large percentage of Americans have or will experience an emotional disorder (Hersen & Van Hasselt, 1994), it is clear that regardless of where they are employed, helpers today *will* be working with some clients who have serious emotional problems or have been given a diagnosis for treatment purposes and/or for legal reasons (see Exercise 8.3). Although defining "abnormality" is still controversial, the use of diagnoses must be addressed by human service professionals today (Fong, 1995; Hohenshil, 1994; Hinkle, 1994a, 1994b). Such classification systems offer a mechanism with which various types of mental health professionals can talk to one another in a similar "diagnostic" language, can understand clients, and can find the best treatment strategies.

EXERCISE 8.3   Diagnosis and Medication: Helpful or Problematic?

In small groups discuss the individuals listed below. Do you believe that a diagnosis hurts or helps each person? Why or why not? Also discuss whether you believe medication is part of the problem or the solution to the problem.

- Tenesha is in the fifth grade and has been assessed as having a conduct disorder and attention deficit disorder with hyperactivity (ADHD). Tenesha takes Ritalin to help her with her attention deficit disorder. Tenesha's mother has a panic disorder and is taking antianxiety medication. Her father is bipolar and taking lithium. It is written into Tenesha's Individualized Education Plan that she should see Jill for individual counseling and for group counseling.
- John is mentally retarded and lives in a group home. He generally has a happy attitude toward life; however, once in a while he "loses it" and has an angry outburst. A few times he almost harmed one of his counselors or one of the other group members. Although behavioral strategies to deal with his outbursts have been tried, they have not been very successful. Thus, he has been placed on medication to assist him in controlling his anger. Everyone, including John, seems more at peace since he started his medication.
- Eduard goes daily to the day treatment center at the local mental health center. He seems fairly coherent and generally in good spirits. He has been hospitalized for schizophrenia on numerous occasions and now takes Haldol and Cogentin to relieve his symptoms. He admits to Jordana, one of his counselors, that when he doesn't take his medication he believes that computers have consciousness and are conspiring throughout the World Wide Web to take over the world. His insurance company pays for his treatment. He will not receive treatment unless Jordana writes his diagnosis on the insurance form.

The *DSM-IV-TR:* A Brief Overview

Derived from the Greek words *dia* (apart) and *gnosis* (to perceive or to know), the term *diagnosis* refers to the process of making an assessment of an individual from an outside, or objective viewpoint (Hersen & Van Hasselt, 1994, p. 6). Although attempts to classify mental disorders have been made since the turn of the century, only in 1952 did the American Psychiatric Association publish the first comprehensive diagnosis system called the *Diagnostic and Statistical Manual of Mental Disorders* (DSM-I). The DSM has been revised numerous times over the years, with the latest edition being the DSM-IV-TR (American Psychiatric Association, 2000; Hinkle, 1994a, b). Although the DSM-IV-TR has its critics (e.g., Wakefield, 1992), it has become the most widespread and accepted diagnostic classification system of emotional disorders. Offering a classification system that is based on five domains, the DSM-IV-TR is a called a multiaxial diagnostic system. Following are very brief descriptions of the five axes. A more in-depth overview of the disorders described in Axes I and II can be found in Appendix D. Try your hand at diagnosing disorders with Exercise 8.4

BOX 8.1   Axis I Disorders

Disorders Usually First Diagnosed in Infancy, Childhood, or Adolescence (excluding Mental Retardation, which is diagnosed on Axis II)

Delirium, Dementia, and Amnestic and Other Cognitive Disorders

Mental Disorders due to a General Medical Condition

Substance-Related Disorders

Schizophrenia and Other Psychotic Disorders

Mood Disorders

Anxiety Disorders

Somatoform Disorders

Factitious Disorders

Dissociative Disorders

Sexual and Gender Disorders

Eating Disorders

Sleep Disorders

Impulse-Control Disorders Not Elsewhere Classified

Adjustment Disorders

Other Conditions That May be a Focus of Clinical Attention.

EXERCISE 8.4   Diagnosing Axis I Disorders

After reading this section and the longer description of the Axis I diagnoses in Appendix D, and using the DSM-IV-TR as your aid, have a student in the class role-play an Axis I disorder. Using the criteria listed in the DSM-IV-TR, try to diagnose the disorder. You may want to role-play a series of Axis I disorders.

Axis I: Clinical Disorders. Other Conditions That May Be a Focus of Clinical Attention   This axis includes all mental health disorders except for those classified as Axis II Disorders (Personality Disorders or Mental Retardation). Box 8.1 lists Axis I Disorders (American Psychiatric Association, 2000, p. 28). Exercise 8.4 allows you to experience the process of diagnosing one of these disorders.

Axis II: Personality Disorders. Mental Retardation   Axis II disorders are notably different from Axis I disorders because they tend to show "an enduring pattern of inner experience and behavior that deviates markedly from the expectation of the individual's culture, is pervasive and inflexible, has an onset in adolescence or early adulthood, is stable over time, and leads to distress or impairment" (American Psychiatric Association, 2000, p. 685).

BOX 8.2   Axis II Disorders

Cluster A:
   Paranoid Personality Disorder
   Schizoid Personality Disorder
   Schizotypal Personality Disorder

Cluster B:
   Antisocial Personality Disorder
   Borderline Personality Disorder
   Histrionic Personality Disorder
   Narcissistic Personality Disorder

Cluster C:
   Avoidant Personality Disorder
   Dependent Personality Disorder
   Obsessive-Compulsive Personality Disorder

EXERCISE 8.5   Diagnosing Axis II Disorders

After reading this section and the longer description of the Axis II diagnoses in Appendix D, and using the DSM-IV-TR as your aid, have a student in the class role-play one of the personality disorders. Using the criteria listed in the DSM-IV-TR, try to identify the disorder. You may want to role-play a few of the personality disorders.

There are 11 personality disorders, 10 of which are grouped under three clusters with the final disorder, Personality Disorder Not Otherwise Specified, being a separate category. Cluster A describes disorders in which the individual appears odd or eccentric. Cluster B describes those disorders in which individuals often exhibit behaviors that are emotional, dramatic, or erratic; and Cluster C delineates disorders in which individuals often seem fearful or anxious (American Psychiatric Association, 2000). The specific disorders are listed in Box 8.2

Exercise 8.5 gives you practice in diagnosing Axis II disorders.

Axis III: General Medical Conditions Axis III provides the clinician with the opportunity to report relevant medical conditions of the client. If the medical condition is clearly related to the cause or worsening of a mental disorder, then the medical condition is listed on both Axis I and/or Axis III. If the medical condition is not a cause of the mental disorder but will affect overall treatment of the individual, then it is listed only on Axis III. An example of an Axis III medical condition that could be a cause of an Axis I diagnosis would

> **EXERCISE 8.6   Diagnosing Medical Conditions**
>
> Have one or more of the role-play clients from Exercise 8.4 or 8.5 role-play a medical condition listed in DSM-IV-TR. Identify the medical condition in DSM-IV-TR and write out the Axis I, Axis II, and Axis III diagnoses. Make sure that the medical condition is listed twice if it is a factor in the Axis I or Axis II diagnosis.

be the development of heart disease that would cause an adjustment disorder. In this case, the heart disease would be noted along with the adjustment disorder on Axis I as well as separately on Axis III. The *International Classification of Diseases,* 9th revision (ICD-9-CM), is used to code the Axis III medical condition, an abbreviated form of which is found in the DSM-IV-TR. Below is an example of a medical condition listed on Axis I and III.

Axis I: Adjustment Disorder with Depressed Mood as a response to congestive heart failure (309.0)

Axis III: Failure, Congestive Heart (428.0)

On the other hand, if an individual had a sleep disorder and subsequently developed acute prostatitis (infection of the prostate), which worsens but was not the original cause of the sleep disorder, it would be written as

Axis I: Narcolepsy (347)

Axis III: Prostatitis (618.9)

If there is no Axis III diagnosis, then a notation of "Axis III: None" is listed. Exercise 8.6 will give you practice in identifying associated medical conditions.

Axis IV: Psychosocial and Environmental Problems Psychosocial or environmental problems that affect the diagnosis, treatment, and prognosis of mental disorders as listed on Axes I and II are noted on Axis IV. Generally, such problems will only be listed on Axis IV, but in those cases where such stressors may be a prime cause of the mental disorder, a reference should be made to them on Axis I or Axis II. General categories of psychosocial and environmental problems include the following: problems with one's primary support group, problems related to the social environment, educational problems, occupational problems, housing problems, economic problems, problems with access to health care services, and problems related to interaction with the legal system/crime. An example of an Axis IV diagnosis might include

Axis IV: Job Loss.

With Exercise 8.7 you can begin working with these diagnoses.

EXERCISE 8.7   Diagnosing Psychosocial and Environmental Problems

Have the role-play client(s) from Exercise 8.6 continue to role-play, or select different students, but each should role-play psychosocial and/or environmental problems. Identify the condition in DSM-IV-TR and write out the Axis I, Axis II, Axis III, and Axis IV diagnoses. Make sure that the psychosocial and environmental problem is listed twice if it is a factor in the Axis I or Axis II diagnosis.

EXERCISE 8.8   Using the GAF Scale

Continue with the role-play(s) from Exercise 8.7 or select other students and determine a GAF score for the client. You may need to probe the client to make an accurate assessment of the score. Have each student in the class do this alone, and then compare your scores with one another.

Axis V: Global Assessment of Functioning (GAF)   Axis V is a scale used by the clinician to assess the overall functioning of the client and is based on his or her psychological, social, and occupational functioning. The GAF scale ranges from very severe to superior functioning, and a score of 0 means there is inadequate information to make a judgment (see Appendix E). In giving a GAF rating, the clinician can report current functioning, the highest functioning within the past year, or any other relevant GAF ratings based on the uniqueness of the situation (see Exercise 8.8).

Making a Diagnosis

The DSM-IV-TR offers decision trees to assist the clinician in making what's called a differential diagnosis. Thus, if one is considering two or more diagnoses that share similar symptoms, the decision tree walks the helper through a series of steps designed to assist him or her in choosing the most appropriate one. It is possible to have more than one Axis I and Axis II diagnosis and in those cases the additional diagnosis should be reported. A typical multiaxial assessment may look something like the following:

Axis I   309.0 Adjustment Disorder with Depressed Features

Axis II   301.82 Avoidant Personality Disorder

Axis III   No Diagnosis

Axis IV   Divorce

Axis V   GAF = 60 (current) 75 (highest in past year)

Exercise 8.9 lets you apply your diagnostic skill with a case study.

EXERCISE 8.9   Using the Five Axes of DSM-IV-TR

Examine the cases of Gloria, David, Jason, and/or Kenny in Appendix F. As well as you can, and using the information that can be found in this chapter and Appendix D, describe each of them on the five axes of DSM-IV-TR.

**EXERCISE 8.10   How Medication Has Helped or Hurt
                 People You Know**

As you discuss each of the classifications of psychotropic medications listed below, share with the class your experience of individuals you know who have either benefited from or been harmed by the use of medication. If you wish, discuss your own use of medication for a mental health problem.

PSYCHOTROPIC MEDICATIONS

Today, a host of medications can be used as adjuncts to counseling in the treatment of many disorders (Schatzberg & Nemeroff, 1998). Ten or 20 years ago, medication was used to treat only severe forms of psychological disorders. With the increase in the types of medications available and the lessening of side effects, medications are now prescribed for almost any kind of psychological problem. Research indicates that medication in conjunction with counseling is more effective than counseling alone in the treatment of depression and other ailments (Conte, Plutchik, Wild, & Karasu, 1986; Norden, 1996), so medication should often be considered as an adjunct to treatment. Many if not most human service professionals today are working with clients who are taking some medication to assist them with emotional problems. What is your experience with psychotropic medication? (See Exercise 8.10.)

Commonly, psychotropic medication has been classified into five groups: antipsychotics, antimanics, antidepressants, antianxiety agents, and stimulants (National Institute of Mental Health, 1995; Donlon, Schaffer, Ericson, Rockwell, & Schaffer, 1983). Following is a brief overview of these five groups. A detailed listing can be found in Appendix G.

Antipsychotics

Antipsychotic drugs are used in treating all types of psychoses and occasionally bipolar disorder, depression with psychotic features, paranoid disorders, and delirium and dementia (Donlon et al., 1983; Marder & Van Putten, 1996; Raskind, 1996). Antipsychotics can dramatically alter the course of treatment for an individual who is having an acute psychotic episode. This is important, for the quicker an individual can recover, the greater the likelihood that future psychotic episodes will not occur. Although antipsychotic medications can assist an individual to live a more normal life, they are often not a "cure." As a number of side effects may occur with many of the medications, antipsychotic drugs such as Thorazine, Haldol, and Risperdal must be carefully prescribed.

Antimanic Medications

In the early 1950s, lithium was found to be an effective treatment for bipolar disorder (then called manic-depression). Lithium seems to act particularly well in lessening the effects of manic symptoms. For individuals who take lithium, the level of drug in the system has to be assessed through a blood test. Too much lithium can cause severe side effects and too little will be ineffective in treatment. Like the antipsychotics, lithium can produce a number of undesirable side effects, although they are generally viewed as less serious than those of the antipsychotic medications. For individuals who don't respond well to lithium, a number of anticonvulsant medications and some benzodiazepines (antianxiety drugs) have been helpful in treating manic episodes (McElroy & Keck, 1996).

Antidepressants

The last 15 years have seen the widespread use of antidepressants called selective serotonin reuptake inhibitors (SSRIs) (Norden, 1996; Tollefson, 1996). The SSRIs have been called miracle drugs by some due to their limited side effects and often dramatic results (Kramer, 1997). Consequently, such drugs as Prozac, Paxil, Luvox, and Zoloft have very quickly become commonplace in American society. In addition to acting beneficially on depression, SSRIs also show promise in treating obsessive-compulsive disorder, panic disorder, some forms of schizophrenia, eating disorders, alcoholism, obesity, and some sleep disorders. Along with the SSRIs, a number of "atypical" antidepressants have also shown promise in the treatment of depression. Some of these include Serzone, Effexor, Wellbutrin, and Remeron.

Antianxiety Medications

The use of modern-day antianxiety agents started with the discovery of Librium, which came on the market in 1960 (Ballenger, 1996). Today, benzodiazepines, such as Valium, Librium, and Xanax, are frequently used in conjunction with psychotherapy for generalized anxiety disorders as they have a calming effect on the individual. Benzodiazepines have also been shown to be helpful in reducing stress, for insomnia, and in management of alcohol withdrawal (Nishino, Mignot, & Dement, 1996). However, tolerance of and dependence on benzodiazepines can occur, and there is a potential for overdose on these medications.

EXERCISE 8.11   Using Psychotropic Medications

In small groups, make an argument for and against the use of each of the five broad categories of drugs. Discuss your arguments in class.

Stimulants

Over the years, amphetamines were used, mostly unsuccessfully, as a diet aid, as an antidepressant, and to relieve the symptoms of sleepiness. However, during the 1950s amphetamines were found to have a "paradoxical effect" in many children diagnosed with attention deficit disorder with hyperactivity (ADHD); it seemed to calm them down and help them focus. Today, the use of stimulants in the treatment of attention deficit disorder is widespread, with the three most common drugs being Ritalin, Cylert, and Dexedrine (Fawcett, & Busch, 1996). Stimulants have also been successful in treating narcolepsy, and are somewhat successful in treating residual attention deficit disorder in adults. Exercise 8.11 probes the pros and cons of psychotropic drugs.

Final Thoughts on Psychotropic Medications

Psychopharmacology has come a long way since the 1950s when the first "modern" psychotropic medications were introduced. Increasingly, medications are used for a wide array of disorders and are more effective and have fewer side effects than in the past. As psychological disorders become better understood, new and even more effective medications can be developed. The human service professional will increasingly need to know the kinds of medications that exist, how they are used in treating mental health problems, and how to refer clients to medical personnel who can prescribe such medications.

CASE REPORT WRITING

Problems associated with writing and reading mental health records are well worth our attention. . . . more and more people are entering in an increasing number of mental health care delivery systems. At the same time, growing numbers of problems are coming to be defined as mental disorders. Consequently, an increasing number of people are writing and reading mental health records for an increasing number of purposes. (Reynolds, Mair, & Fischer, 1995, p. 1)

With the changing times has come a greater emphasis on the importance of accurate record keeping. Although this can be taken to extremes; there is no question that good case records can (Kleinke, 1994; Neukrug, 1999a)

- be used in court to show adequate client care took place.
- assist helpers in conceptualizing client problems and making diagnoses.
- help determine whether clients have made progress.
- be useful when obtaining supervision.
- assist the helper in remembering what the client said.
- sometimes be mandated by insurance companies and government agencies in order to approve the treatment being given to clients, and in this age of accountability.
- be a determining factor for which agencies will receive funding.

Types of Case Report Writing

Today, depending on the agency, many kinds of case report writing will be required. These include daily case notes, intake summaries, quarterly summaries, and summaries for companies, students' individual education plans, vocational rehabilitation planning, referrals to other clinicians, and termination, to name just a few.

In recording case reports, a lucky helper may work at an agency in which there is a secretary who will type dictation. However, many agencies ask helpers to type their own notes directly into the computer (Nurius & Hudson, 1989a, 1989b; Tiedeman, 1983). Or, as in the past, many helpers today are still asked to keep notes in the tried-and-true fashion of writing them out.

Probably, the minimum information that should be included in records are the name of the client, the date, major facts noted during contact, progress made toward achieving client goals, and the helper's signature. Other headings may include demographic information (e.g., date of birth, address, phone, date of interview), reason for report, family background, other pertinent background information (e.g., health information, vocational history, history of adjustment issues/emotional problems/mental illness), mental status, assessment results, diagnosis, and summary, conclusions, and recommendations (see example of report in Appendix H). Although all of these headings are important, the mental status deserves special attention as it is often a misunderstood area of the case report.

Mental Status The mental status exam is often completed by the helper and is a statement of (1) how the client presents himself or herself (appearance), (2) the client's ability to think clearly (thought disturbance), (3) the client's feeling state (affect), and (4) the client's memory state and orientation to the world (cognition). Generally, a client's mental status can be obtained through the clinical interview. Below is an abbreviated definition of each of these four areas (for a more complete example, see the mental status exam in

> **EXERCISE 8.12   Writing a Mental Status Report**
>
> Find a partner and first have one person role-play a seriously impaired client while the other tries to assess, as a helper, the client's mental status. Then write a mental status report. After the first role-play, switch roles and have the second helper assess and write the mental status report. Use the mental status report section of the case report in Appendix H as a model. When you have finished, discuss the following issues in class:
>
> 1. How difficult was it to assess a client's mental status?
> 2. What would have helped you in your assessment?
> 3. What questions might help you in assessing all four areas of the client's mental status? Write them on the board and note them for future use.

the case report, Appendix H). (Note: For a fuller description of the mental status exam, see Carson, 2000.)

1. *Appearance:* This is a statement about how the client looks, any negative attitudes the client might present, the client's mode of speech (e.g., labored, rapid), eye contact, hygiene, posture, and other obvious observable activities.

2. *Affect:* This is a statement about the feeling state of the client. The affect is the immediate feelings the client is expressing (e.g., sad, happy, depressed, angry) whereas mood refers to the long-term feelings of the client. Affect can be flat, appropriate, full, or labile (all over the place).

3. *Thought disturbance:* This is a statement about the thought processes of the client and whether the client is delusional (e.g., client thinks he is Jesus Christ) or has auditory or visual hallucinations. A client's thought process may include loose associations (thinking is all over the place), or tangential thinking (ideas that seem to go off on a tangent), or circumstantial thinking (ideas that seem to take forever but go around in a circle to get back to where they started). Clients also may have suicidal or homicidal ideation.

4. *Cognition:* This part of the mental status exam looks at whether the client knows what time it is, where he or she is, and who he or she is (whether the client is oriented to time, place, and person). It also assesses the client's short- and long-term memory, general intellectual functioning, and ability to make sound judgments and be insightful.

In Exercise 8.12, you have the opportunity to write a mental status report.

Writing Case Notes

Any written information about a client needs to be objective and should be based on observable behavior, not opinion. Remember that what a helper writes could be subpoenaed for use in court and a helper could be held liable for his or her statements. Therefore, writing from an objective, dispassionate

---

EXERCISE 8.13   Writing a Case Report

Using the information you gathered in Exercise 8.12, or after interviewing a
different student, write a case report using some or all of the suggested
categories listed below. Keep your case report to three pages, single-spaced.
You might want to use the model of a case report that is located in Appendix
H to guide you. When the case report is complete, share it with others in small
groups to gain feedback, or hand it in to your instructor who will review it and
give you feedback.

Possible Categories for Case Report

1. Demographic Information (e.g., Date of Birth, Address, Phone, Date of
   Interview)
2. Reason for Report
3. Family Background
4. Other Pertinent Background Information (e.g., Health Information,
   Vocational History, History of Adjustment Issues/Emotional Problems/Mental
   Illness)
5. Mental Status
6. Assessment Results
7. Diagnosis
8. Summary, Conclusions, and Recommendations

---

point of view is essential when keeping case notes. Generally, only the third
person should be used in referring to the client. For example, it would be better to say, "Family information was gathered from Jim," than "I collected family information from Jim." Any subjective information that is gathered from
the client should be noted as such. To assist in this, begin subjective statements
with the following phrases such as, "It seems that . . .," "Jim noted
that . . .," "It appears that . . .," "Jim reported that . . .," "Claire related
that . . .," and "Claire recounted that . . ."

When writing case notes helpers should try not to side with their clients,
portray sexist attitudes, use significant amounts of psychological jargon, or
make statements expressing their own values or opinions (unless the helper's
opinions are called for, as when a court is asking for it or the helper is making
a diagnosis). Also, write the report so that other mental health professionals
would readily understand it. Finally, of course, use good grammar. See Appendix H for an example of a case report, then try writing your own using
the directions in Exercise 8.13.

Security of Record Keeping

Generally, clients have the right to have information they share with the helper
kept confidential. However, there are some exceptions to this rule: (1) if your
employer (e.g. agency administrator) requests information from a helper regarding a client, (2) if a helper shares client information with a supervisor as a
means of assisting the helper in his or her work with the client, (3) if the court

---

How Secure Are Records?

Unfortunately, I have found that helpers sometimes forget how easily client records can be misplaced or the information in them made too readily available to the public. The following true stories highlight the ways that information in records can be mishandled and stress the importance of keeping records secure and confidential.

1. When I worked as an outpatient therapist at a comprehensive mental health center, a client of another therapist had apparently appropriated his records that had been left "lying around." Because the therapist's records were written in "psychologese" using diagnostic language, the client was understandably quite upset by what he found. He would periodically call the emergency services at night and read his records over the phone to the emergency worker while making fun of the language used in the records.

2. When I was in my doctoral program, we were reviewing an intellectual test assessment of an adolescent that had been done a number of years earlier. Suddenly, one of the students in the class yelled out, "That's me!" Apparently, although there was no identifying name on the report, he recognized it as describing him (he had been given a copy of the report previously).

These two examples show the importance of keeping client information confidential and secure.

---

subpoenas a helper's records, (4) if a client gives permission, in writing, to share information with others, or (5) in most cases, if a parent requests information about his or her child. Written client records need to be kept in secured places such as locked file cabinets and nonaccessible computer disks. Clerical help need to understand the importance of confidentiality when working with records. Some agencies have clerical staff sign statements acknowledging that they understand the importance of the confidentiality of records.

Clients' Rights to Records

Increasingly, clients have been given the approval of the courts to obtain copies of reports about them that are kept on file in schools, hospitals, and clinics (Wicks, 1993; Swenson, 1997). Also, it has generally been assumed that parents have the right to view records of their children (C. Borstein, attorney, personal communication, February 20, 2001). Case report writers should be aware of this access prior to writing reports (Wicks, 1977).

In terms of federal law, the Freedom of Information Act of 1974 allows individuals access to records maintained by a federal agency that contain personal information about the individual. Similarly, the Buckley Amendment of 1974, otherwise known as the Family Education Rights and Privacy Act (FERPA), assures parents the right to access their children's educational records (Committee on Government Operations, 1991).

On a more practical level, a client rarely asks to see his or her records. However, if a client did make such a request, I would first attempt to talk with the client about what is written in the records. If this was not satisfactory to him or her, I would then suggest that I might write a summary of the records. However, if a client steadfastly stated a desire to view his or her records, I believe that this is his or her right and I would give that client a copy of the record.

MANAGING AND DOCUMENTING CLIENT CONTACT HOURS

Managing Client Hours

Human service professionals often find themselves with very large caseloads and are expected to meet with all of their clients in a manner that assures sound clinical treatment. With large numbers of clients, it is unfortunately sometimes easy to not follow-up when appointments are missed, to arrange meeting with clients at intervals that are shorter than are clinically appropriate, or to even forget about arranging appointment times for some clients. To assure that clients are afforded appropriate treatment, it is essential that human service professionals find a mechanism that assures proper management of client contact hours. This sometimes takes some creative activities, such as running special groups (e.g., medication review groups), working additional evening hours to meet with clients who cannot make it in during the day, and using day planners and palm pilots (electronic hand held organizers).

Documenting Client Contact Hours

Today, it has become important for helpers to document contact hours, as reimbursement by insurance companies, as well as local, state, and federal funding agencies, is often based on clear records of these hours. Thus, most agencies today have some mechanism for recording helper/client hours. This can be done by hand on a simple grid; but increasingly, documentation is completed with the use of computer software specifically developed for this purpose. Exercise 8.14 helps you determine how client hours should be recorded.

EXERCISE 8.14   Documenting Client Hours

On your own or in small groups develop a sample grid you could use to document client hours. What information do you need to include? When you have finished, share your grid with others in class.

MONITORING, EVALUATING, AND DOCUMENTING PROGRESS TOWARD CLIENT GOALS

All human service professionals should monitor client progress toward goals to assure that the client is progressing and feels cared about in the process. If goals are not being met, they need to be reviewed and adjusted accordingly.

The documentation of progress toward goals is increasingly being reviewed by funding agencies. In fact, some funding agencies today will not renew funding if documentation and progress are not shown. The simplest way to document progress toward goals is to make a note in the client's chart. Innovative human service professionals can create charts and graphs to visually document client progress. Finally, the Global Assessment of Functioning (GAF) scale of DSM-IV-TR is increasingly being used as one measurement of progress toward goals and treatment success.

MAKING REFERRALS

There are many reasons to refer a client to another professional. A client may be referred as a part of the treatment plan, because the professional is leaving the agency, because the professional feels incompetent to work with the client, or because the client has reached his or her goals and is ready to move on to another form of treatment. In any case, the manner in which the referral is made is very important to continued client progress. In referrals, professionals should do the following:

1. Discuss the reason for making the referral with the client and obtain his or her approval.
2. Obtain, in writing, permission to discuss anything about the client with another professional, even if simply sharing the client's name with another professional.
3. Monitor the client's progress with the other professional.
4. Assure that confidentiality of client information is maintained in the referral process.

Practice referral making with Exercise 8.15.

EXERCISE 8.15   Making Referrals

Find a fellow student and have one role-play a helper while the other role-plays a client. Choose one of the reasons listed above for why a helper might refer a client and role-play a situation in which such a referral is to take place. Reflect on how it feels to make a referral of a client. Share your feelings in small groups or with the class.

FOLLOW-UP

Follow-up, another important function of case management, can be completed by a phone call, by a letter, by an elaborate survey of clients, or by other ways. It can be done a few days to a few weeks after the relationship has ended and serves many purposes (Hutchins & Cole, 1992; Kleinke, 1994; Neukrug, 2000):

1. It functions as a check to see whether clients would like to return for counseling or be referred to a different helper.
2. It allows the helper to assess whether change has been maintained.
3. It gives the helper the opportunity to determine which counseling techniques have been most successful.
4. It offers an opportunity to reinforce client change.
5. It allows the helper to evaluate services provided to the client.

TIME MANAGEMENT

With ever-increasing caseloads and demands placed on the helper, time management has become crucial if the helper is to avoid burnout. Many time management systems have been created to help working professionals manage their heavy caseloads. Although this text does not delve into these different systems, addressing time management concerns is important to all human service professionals.

SUMMARY

The chapter examined case management, which includes (1) treatment planning: assessing needs and developing goals, (2) diagnosis, (3) monitoring the use of psychotropic drugs, (4) case report writing, (5) managing and documenting client contact hours, (6) monitoring, evaluating, and documenting progress toward client goals, (7) making referrals, (8) follow-up, and (9) time management.

Treatment planning involves both an assessment of client needs and the development of client goals. Assessing client needs can be done with the clinical interview, testing, observation, client self-assessment, assessment of client by others, and a review of client records. The development of client goals, a collaborative process, grows out of assessment. Goals should be attainable, changed when necessary, and monitored and reinforced. New goals can be established as former goals are reached, but a good helping professional also knows when the client should stop trying to attain goals.

The importance of diagnosis was discussed, mainly in terms of the five axes of DSM-IV-TR. These include Axis I: Clinical Disorders and Other Conditions That May be a Focus of Clinical Attention; Axis II: Personality Disorders and Mental Retardation; Axis III: General Medical Conditions; Axis IV: Psychosocial and Environmental Problems; and Axis V: The Global Assessment of Functioning (GAF) Scale.

The modern-day use of psychotropic medication is broad, with medications now prescribed for almost any kind of psychological problem. The classification of psychopharmacological drugs was examined, primarily these five groups: antipsychotics, antimanics, antidepressants, antianxiety agents, and stimulants.

The next case management activity discussed was managing and writing case reports. Particular attention was paid to how to write a mental status report. Specific ethical, professional, and legal issues related to case notes were explored such as the security of records, clients' rights to records, and confidentiality of written records.

Other issues in case management that received attention were managing and documenting client contact hours; monitoring, evaluating, and documenting progress toward client goals; how and when to make referrals; how to follow-up with clients; and how to manage time when working with many clients.

Case management has become an increasingly complex process occurring throughout all the stages of the helping relationship. It needs to be addressed carefully by all human service professionals regardless of where they work.

SPECIAL INTEGRATION
OF CASE MANAGEMENT EXERCISE

1. Interview a client and incorporate the following case management procedures in your interview: treatment planning, diagnosis, referral for medication, and case report writing including mental status exam and report.

 ## INFOTRAC COLLEGE EDITION

1. Pick a diagnosis from the "DSM-IV-TR" (you may need to use the keyword "DSM-IV") categories and research it in more detail.

2. Examine how "psychopharmacology" is used within a treatment category of your choice.

3. Research any of the case management categories highlighted in this chapter.

9

Multicultural Counseling

Issues and Techniques

INTRODUCTION

Cross-cultural counseling relationships have become more common in today's helping situations, yet counseling does not always seem to work for minorities. To help reverse this trend, the chapter offers an existential model for understanding culturally diverse clients and highlights the importance to helpers of having appropriate beliefs and attitudes, such as knowledge of their own cultural backgrounds, biases, stereotypes, and values. Helpers also need knowledge of different ethnic and cultural groups as well as specific skills if they are to work successfully with culturally diverse clients.

The second part of the chapter suggests ways to work with individuals from different ethnic and racial groups, people from diverse religious backgrounds, women, men, gays and lesbians, individuals who are HIV positive, the homeless and the poor, older persons, the mentally ill, and individuals with disabilities.

WHY MULTICULTURAL COUNSELING?

The Changing Face of America

America is the most diverse country in the world and is becoming increasingly more so (Whitfield, 1994). Today, over one-third of the population is composed of racial and ethnic minorities, and midway through this century

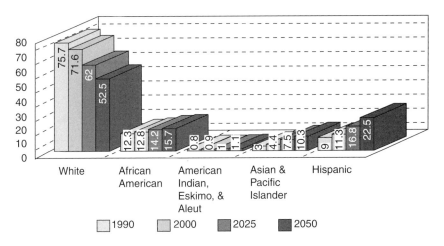

FIGURE 9.1 Percentage of Population by Race/Culture over Time

minorities will constitute almost 50% of the American population (U.S. Department of Commerce, 1996). By mid-century, we will see an increase in Native Americans, from 0.8% to 1.2%; Asian and Pacific Islanders, from 3% to 10%; Hispanics, from 9% to 23%; African Americans from 12% to 16%; and a decrease in white Americans, from 76% to 53% (see Figure 9.1).

These changing demographics are a function of several factors: birth rates are higher within minority populations; most immigrants no longer come from Western countries; and immigration rates are the highest in American history. The great majority of immigrants are now Asian (34%) or Hispanic (34%), compared to past immigrants who were mostly white European; and there is a greater tendency among all immigrants to want to assert their cultural heritage rather than be swallowed up by the Western-based American culture.

Changes in the racial, ethnic, and cultural backgrounds of Americans bring changes in the religious composition of the country as well (National Opinion Research Center, 1991). As increased numbers of Asians, Hispanics, and Middle Easterners arrive at our shores, we find religions that were previously rare in America. But diversity in religion is not only brought by immigrants. Although America is largely Christian, diversity in Christianity is greater than ever. From a multitude of Protestant faiths, to Roman Catholics who are increasingly varied in their beliefs, to Eastern Orthodox, Mormons, Christian Scientists, Seventh Day Adventists, Amish, Mennonites, and on and on, the Christian religion in America is a religious mosaic in and of itself.

In addition to the changing ethnic, cultural, and religious diversity, there are changes in sex-role identity as well. The "macho" male is no longer considered a model for maleness while expectations concerning the woman's role in the workplace and as a child care provider have changed dramatically. There is also an increased awareness of the gay and lesbian culture. Whereas in the past many homosexuals felt a need to hide their sexual orientation for fear of discrimination, today an increasing number of gays and lesbians are "coming out."

Changes in federal, state, and local laws, as well as a gradual move toward more tolerance of differentness in our culture, have given many Americans an increased sensitivity to and awareness of a number of special groups, including the physically challenged, older persons, the homeless and the poor, individuals who are HIV positive, and the mentally ill. Changing demographics in the country make it increasingly important for helpers to make sure that their counseling approach works with a wide variety of clients. Unfortunately, this has not always been the case. Exercise 9.1 will help you explore your values toward diverse clients.

Counseling Is Not Working for a Large Segment of the Population

If you were distrustful of helpers, confused about the counseling process, or felt worlds apart from the helper you were seeing, would you want to continue in the helping relationship? Assuredly not. Unfortunately, this is the state of affairs for many minority clients (Steward, Neil, Jo, Hill, & Baden, 1998). In fact, when minority clients work with majority helpers there is a strong possibility that the helper will (1) minimize the impact of social forces on the client, (2) interpret cultural differences as psychopathological issues, and (3) misdiagnosis the client (Mwaba & Pedersen, 1990).

Counseling is not productive for many clients from diverse backgrounds. A large body of evidence shows that minority clients are frequently misunderstood, often misdiagnosed, find therapy less helpful than their majority counterparts, attend therapy at lower rates than majority clients, and tend to terminate therapy more quickly than majority clients (Cole & Pilisuk, 1976; Copeland, 1983; Garretson, 1993; Shipp, 1983; Lee & Mixson, 1995; Poston, Craine, & Atkinson, 1991; Solomon, 1992; Wilson & Stith, 1991). In addition, clients from cultural backgrounds different from that of their helper may experience the helping relationship more negatively than if the helper is of the same culture (Atkinson, 1985; Atkinson, Poston, Furlong, & Mercado, 1989). It is understandable that minority clients are underrepresented at mental health centers (Sue & Sue, 1990).

Why is counseling not working for a good segment of our population? Some have suggested the following reasons (Midgette & Meggert, 1991; Sodowsky & Taffe, 1991; Solomon, 1992; Yutrzenka, 1995):

1. *The melting pot myth.* Many see this country as a melting pot, or blending of cultural diversity. However, this is *not* the experience of many minority clients who find themselves on the fringe of American culture and cannot relate to many of the values and beliefs held by the majority. Helpers who idealistically believe we are all the same may turn off the minority client who has not had this "melting pot" experience. Probably, the view of America as a *cultural mosaic* that has a myriad of diverse values and customs is a more accurate conceptualization of the country today.

EXERCISE 9.1   A Loving Story

While on a business trip, Lovey's significant other, Fine, is called to active duty to fight a war in another part of the world. Fine leaves for base camp before Lovey can get home. Wanting one last night with Fine, Lovey approaches the base commander, March, and begs March to let Lovey spend one last night with Fine. March, who is a national hero for saving POWs, explains that this is against the rules and to break the rules for one person is not right. March, who silently struggles with constant severe back pain from saving the POWs, goes on to state that "under the right circumstances, rules could be broken." Realizing March is making a pass, Lovey says "no way," and walks off discouraged.

Lovey next approaches Friend, who reminds Lovey that Lovey has "slept around" and then states "What's the big deal about sleeping with one more person?" Thinking that Friend has a point, Lovey returns to March, flirts, and eventually makes a deal to trade sex for one last night with Fine. After sex, Lovey is allowed to see Fine. Believing in honest relationships, Lovey tells Fine the whole story, at which point Fine becomes enraged and strikes Lovey. Feeling guilt-ridden and dejected, Fine leaves, later attempts suicide, and ends up in a psychiatric hospital. Accepting blame as the cause of Fine's suicide attempt, Lovey goes to talk with Dr. Jaime, who explains that Fine's suicide attempt was of Fine's own choosing and that Lovey shouldn't have self-blame.

A. Examining Values as a Function of Gender and Ethnicity
Scoring Your Results: Using the grid below, rate each of the five characters in the story. Place an X under number 1 and across from the name of the person you like most. Then place an X under number 2 and across from the name you like second most, and so forth. Your instructor will then count up all the 1s, 2s, 3s, 4s, and 5s in the class and place them on a master grid on the board.

	1	2	3	4	5
Lovey					
Fine					
March					
Friend					
Dr. Jaime					

(Continued)

EXERCISE 9.1   Continued

Then, as a class, respond to the following questions:

1. What does the distribution tell you about how students in your class view individuals with differing values?
2. Based on the characters' roles, did you assume that certain characters in the story were male and others were female?
3. Consider how you might rate the characters if you changed their gender.
4. If the characters in the story were of differing ethnic, cultural, or religious backgrounds, would you have responded differently to them?
5. If you were in a helping relationship with any of the characters in the story, how would your positive and negative stereotypes affect your work with them?

B. Alternative to the Above Exercise
Instead of having the class complete Exercise A, the instructor will divide the class into six groups and have each group make assumptions about the characters as noted below. Then, using the scoring instructions in "A," collect the aggregate data in each of the six groups and compare the responses of the six different groups. (Feel free to create other groups of different gender and ethnic mixes.)

1. *Group 1 (All characters are white)*
   Lovey is female, Fine is male, March is male, Friend is female, Dr. Jaime is male
2. *Group 2 (All characters are African American)*
   Lovey is female, Fine is male, March is male, Friend is female, Dr. Jaime is male
3. *Group 3 (Female characters are white, male characters are black)*
   Lovey is female, Fine is male, March is male, Friend is female, Dr. Jaime is male
4. *Group 4 (Male characters are white, female characters are black)*
   Lovey is female, Fine is male, March is male, Friend is female, Dr. Jaime is male
5. *Group 5 (All characters are female)*
6. *Group 6 (All characters are male)*

---

2. *Incongruent expectations about the helping relationship.* The Western, particularly American, approach to the helping relationship emphasizes the individual; stresses the expression of feelings; tries to show cause and effect; and encourages self-disclosure, open-mindedness, and insight (see Box 9.1). Because people in many cultures do not place high value on these attributes, the helping relationship often does not meet their expectations. For example, the Asian client who is proud of her ability to restrict her emotions may leave the helping relationship disappointed that her helper has been pushing her to express feelings.

3. *Lack of understanding of social forces.* Helpers often assume that negative feelings are created by the individual, and they overlook the power of social influences. Such helpers will have a difficult time with a client who

---

BOX 9.1 Western Values Stressed in the Helping Relationship

Primary Language: Standard English/some helpers are bilingual

Locus of Control/Locus of Responsibility: Individual/individual

Major Inherent Values: (1) Verbal/emotional/behavioral expressiveness, (2) Openness and intimacy, (3) Linear/cause and effect, (4) Analytical, (5) Self-disclosure

Primary Communication Path: Communication: Client to helper

Mental/Physical Processes: Dichotomous: Mind/body separation

Religion: Neutral (Helpers generally do not support one religious point of view over another)

Gender Focus: Neutral (Nonsexist ideals are stressed)

Focus on Family: (Nuclear family) Helper examines impact of client issues on nuclear family

Adapted from Atkinson, Morten, and Sue (1993); Sue and Sue (1990); Pedersen, Draguns, Lonner, and Trimble (1996); and McGoldrick, Pearce, and Giordano (1996).

---

has been considerably harmed by external factors. For instance, the client who was illegally denied jobs due to his disability may be discouraged when a helper says, "What have *you* done to prevent yourself from obtaining the job?"

4. *Ethnocentric worldview.* Many helpers falsely assume that clients view the world as they do, or believe that when clients present a different worldview, it is an indication of emotional instability or client misunderstanding. For instance, a helper may inadvertently offend a Muslim when she says to her client, "Have a wonderful Christmas."

5. *Ignorance of one's own racist attitudes and prejudices.* When helpers are not in touch with their prejudices, stereotypes, and racist attitudes, they cannot work effectively with minority clients. For instance, the helper who unconsciously believes homosexuality is a disease but states he is accepting of all sexual orientations, may subtly treat a gay client as if there is something wrong with him or her.

6. *Inability to understand cultural differences in the expression of symptomatology.* The helper's lack of knowledge about cultural differences as they relate to the expression of symptoms can harm the helping relationship, resulting in misdiagnosis, mistreatment, and early termination. For instance, whereas many individuals from Western cultures show grief through depression, agitation, and feelings of helplessness, a Mexican might present with somatic complaints.

7. *The unreliability of assessment and research instruments.* Over the years, assessment and research instruments have notoriously been culturally biased. For example, a religious Hispanic, when asked on a personality test if she

"hears voices," might answer "yes," thinking that she "talks to God"— a normal response in her culture. In American culture, talking to God could be interpreted as evidence of schizophrenia. Although Americans might also "talk to God," they have learned to deny "hearing voices" because that implies psychopathology in this culture.

8. *Institutional racism.* Because racism is embedded in society and often unrecognized by many (D'Andrea, 1996), materials used by helpers may be biased. For instance, some DSM-IV-TR diagnoses have been shown to be culturally biased; well-accepted counseling approaches have been practically useless with some minorities; and human services training programs have not, until recently, stressed multicultural issues. No doubt, there are culturally biased statements in this text of which I am not aware.

9. *A counseling process not designed for clients from diverse backgrounds.* Helpers have been accused of wanting to work with young, attractive, verbal, intelligent, and successful clients ("YAVIS"), rather than clients who are quiet, ugly, old, indigent, and dissimilar culturally ("QUOID"). For many culturally diverse clients, the traditional counseling process is not beneficial and can be harmful (Sodowsky & Taffe, 1991; Yutrzenka, 1995). For example, counseling appears to be particularly unsuccessful with low socioeconomic status African Americans, Asian Americans, Hispanics, and American Indians.

Clearly, there is a need for multicultural counseling. In the past few years there has been an outcry by many in the helping professions for greater sensitivity in counseling diverse clients (Baker, 1995; Fukuyama, 1994; Lee, 1994; Sandhu, 1995; Sue, Arredondo, & McDavis, 1992; Sue & Sue, 1990). For culturally different clients, this call to the profession should result in (1) helpers having a better understanding of diversity, (2) helpers being able to make more accurate diagnoses, (3) a decrease in the dropout rate from counseling by minorities, and (4) an increase in satisfaction with the helping process (Quintana & Bernal, 1995).

THE HELPING RELATIONSHIP AND CULTURAL DIVERSITY

A Model for Understanding Culturally Diverse Clients

"Every person is like all persons, like some persons, and like no other person" (paraphrased from Kluckhorn & Murray, cited in Speight, Myers, Cox, & Highlen, 1991, p. 32).

Existentialists have noted that in trying to understand individuals, you need to be aware of an individual's uniqueness (**Eigenwelt**), the common experiences held by groups and cultures (**Mitwelt**), and shared universal experiences

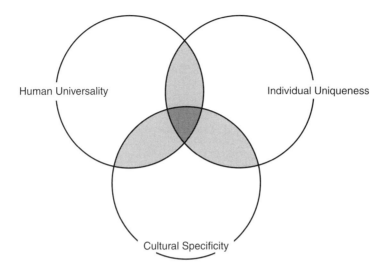

FIGURE 9.2 A Model for Understanding Cultural Diversity
Each sphere represents a unique aspect of the individual. The area
where the spheres overlap is too small to represent the total client. To
understand the client fully we must learn about all three spheres.

SOURCE: From "A Redefinition of Multicultural Counseling," by S. L. Speight, J. Myers, D. F. Fox,
and P. S. Highlen, 1991, *Journal of Counseling and Development, 70,* 29–36. Copyright © 1991.
American Counseling Association. Reprinted by permission. No further reproduction authorized
without permission.

EXERCISE 9.2   Developing a Multicultural Approach to Counseling

Form small groups and discuss your view of the effective cross-cultural helper.
What is different about this helper compared to a helper who cannot work
effectively with culturally different clients? Share your answers with the class,
and have your instructor make a list, on the board, of the qualities of the
effective cross-cultural helper.

(*Umwelt*) (Binswanger, 1962, 1963). Keeping this in mind, you should ask
"How can the helper be effective with culturally different clients?" Using the
above existential framework as a model, you would conclude that each client
has specific issues related to his or her culture, is unique unto himself or herself, and shares universal issues common to all people (Speight et al., 1991,
p. 32) (see Figure 9.2). Each of these spheres represents a unique aspect of the
individual. The area of overlap is so small that the helper must understand all
three spheres if he or she is to truly understand the client. Exercise 9.2 can
help you identify the qualities of an effective multicultural counselor.

Culturally Skilled Professionals: Beliefs and Attitudes, Knowledge, and Skills

A number of authors have stated that to work effectively with clients, culturally skilled mental health professionals must be aware of their attitudes and beliefs toward culturally diverse populations, have a knowledge base that supports their work with diverse clients, and have the necessary skills to help clients with diverse backgrounds (Pedersen et al., 1996; Sue et al., 1992; Sue et al., 1982).

Beliefs and Attitudes Culturally skilled human service professionals have an awareness of their own cultural backgrounds, biases, stereotypes, and values, and such helpers should have the ability to respect differences. Although culturally skilled human service professionals may not hold the same belief system as their clients, they can accept differing worldviews. Being sensitive to differences and knowing one's own cultural biases allow culturally skilled human service processionals to refer a minority client to a professional of the client's own race or culture when a referral will benefit the client.

Knowledge Culturally skilled human service professionals have an awareness of sociopolitical issues in the United States, have knowledge of the barriers that hinder culturally diverse clients from using social service agencies, and possess specific knowledge about clients' cultural or ethnic groups. Such skilled human service professionals have or are willing to gain a knowledge of characteristics of specific cultural, racial, and ethnic groups (for example, personality styles, customs, traditions). At the same time, such human service professionals do not assume that just because clients come from a specific cultural background, they necessarily have these characteristics. In other words, human service professionals have knowledge of the group from which clients come, yet do not make assumptions about clients' ways of being.

Skills Human service professionals who are effective with culturally diverse populations are able to apply generic interviewing and helping skills with culturally diverse populations while being aware of and able to apply specialized interventions that might be effective with specific populations. Related to this, culturally sensitive human service professionals understand the verbal and nonverbal language of clients and can communicate effectively with them.

THE HELPING RELATIONSHIP
WITH SPECIFIC POPULATIONS

While the application of specific helping skills discussed in this text may be beneficial to some clients, they may not be helpful, and even may be harmful to the helping relationship when used with other clients. For instance, many Latin American clients are comfortable with less personal space than other clients and may interpret helper distance as aloofness; a Muslim may consider being touched by the left hand of a helper as obscene as the left hand is seen as unclean and used as an aid in the process of elimination while the right hand is seen as clean and used to eat with; and an African American client may be put off by eye contact from a white helper (Sue & Sue, 1990).

On a broader scale, as a function of a particular culture, some clients may feel defensive with the use of questions, while other clients may feel stonewalled because the helper uses too much empathy. Some clients may feel as though they are being pushed to self-disclose—a quality viewed as a weakness in their culture, while other clients may feel offended that the helper has not allowed them to talk more as their culture is one in which feelings are openly expressed. Clients of some cultures may be embarrassed with helper self-disclosure; for others, such disclosure may bring a helper and client who are from two different cultures closer together.

Clearly, helpers need to have knowledge of the cultural background of the client and how much a specific client's values, beliefs, and customs will play a part in the helping relationship. However, it must also be remembered that each client is unique. For instance, although many Latin American clients may be turned off by too much helper-client personal space, some will not—and may indeed even feel more comfortable. An acculturated African American client may be offended by the intentional *lack* of eye contact from his or her white helper as a result of the helper's false belief that all African Americans would prefer less eye contact from white helpers.

The following section and Exercise 9.3 offer some suggestions for working with select populations. Keep in mind that these are suggestions and that each client is unique.

EXERCISE 9.3   Identifying Counseling Needs of Culturally Different Clients

This exercise can be done individually or in small groups. Below is a select list of culturally different groups. Some individuals from such groups have unique needs in the helping relationship, which are related to their cultural/ethnic background. Identify one or more of the groups listed below and discuss how you think the helping relationship might best work with individuals from that group. Feel free to add other groups to this list.

African Americans	Men	The poor
Diverse religions	Bisexuals	Older persons
Lesbian women	The homeless	Native Americans
Individuals with disabilities	Asians	Gay men
Individuals who are HIV positive	Women	People with mental illness
Hispanics		

Counseling Individuals from Different Ethnic and Racial Groups

Although cultural differences are great among African Americans, Asian Americans, Hispanics, and Native Americans, there are some broad suggestions that can be followed for working with individuals from these and other cultures. Westwood and Ishiyama (1990), Neukrug (1994, 2000), and others note that the following should be attended to when counseling individuals from different cultures.

1. *Encourage clients to speak their own language.* A helper is not necessarily expected to be bilingual, although that would often be a benefit, and referral to a bilingual helper sometimes is appropriate. If a client is bilingual and the helper is not, the helper should make an effort to know meaningful expressions of the client's language.

2. *Learn about the cultural heritage of clients.* Helpers should make sure that they have taken workshops or courses, researched the client's culture in the library, and/or have asked their clients about their cultural heritage.

3. *Assess client's cultural identity.* Try to understand how clients view themselves relative to their culture. For example, a client who has acculturated and has little identification with his or her culture of origin is very different from a client from the same culture who is a new immigrant.

4. *Check the accuracy of clients' nonverbal expression.* Don't assume that nonverbal communication is consistent across cultures. Helpers should ask their clients about their nonverbal expression when in doubt.

5. *Make use of alternate modes of communication.* Because of cross-cultural differences, some clients will be reticent to talk, and for others, English may be a second language that they are hesitant to use for fear of making mistakes. When reasonable, use other modes of communication such as acting, drawing, music, storytelling, or collage making, which may draw out a client.

6. *Encourage clients to bring in culturally significant and personally relevant items.* Helpers should have clients bring in items that will assist the helper to understand them and their culture (e.g., book, photograph, article of significance, culturally meaningful items).

7. *Vary the helping environment.* The helping relationship may be quite unfamiliar territory to a client, and sitting in a small private room might create intense anxiety. Thus, it may be important to explore alternative helping environments to ease clients into the helping relationship (e.g., take a walk, have a cup of coffee at a quiet restaurant, initially meet clients at their home).

8. *Don't jump to conclusions about clients.* Don't fall into the trap of assuming that clients will act in stereotypic ways. Many clients won't match a stereotype.

9. *Know yourself.* Helpers should assess their own biases and prejudices to assure that they will not negatively affect the helping relationship.

10. *Know appropriate skills.* Helpers should take courses and attend workshops, and should keep up with the most recent professional literature to assure that they know the most appropriate helping skills to use and *not use* with clients.

Counseling Individuals from Diverse Religious Backgrounds

In working with any individual it is important to understand his or her religious background, for this may hold the key to understanding the person's underlying values. Some pointers to keep in mind concerning religion and the helping relationship include the following:

1. *Determine the client's religious background early in the helping relationship.* As a basis for future treatment planning, helpers should know the client's religious affiliation. This information can be acquired at the initial interview; however, a helper should be sensitive to any client who may initially resist a discussion of religion.

2. *Ask the client how important religion is in his or her life.* For some clients, religion holds little influence; for others, it is a driving force. In either case, most clients have only a rudimentary understanding of their religious tradition, and helpers should not assume that clients know much about their religion even if they present themselves as deeply religious. Assessment of the part religion plays in a client's life can assist in goal setting and treatment planning.

3. *Assess the client's level of faith development.* Low-stage faith development clients will tend to be more dualistic and concrete (Fowler, 1981). This client works better with a fair amount of structure and firm goals. High-stage faith development clients see the world in complex ways and value many kinds of faith experiences. This client likely would feel more comfortable in a helping relationship that values abstract thinking and self-reflection.

4. *Be careful not to make false assumptions about clients.* Some false assumptions are made when a helper takes a stereotypic view of the client's religion. For instance, some helpers might falsely believe that all Jews keep a kosher home. Another kind of false assumption results when a helper projects his or her religious views onto others. For instance, some Christian helpers may assume that all faiths believe people are born with original sin. In actuality, this is solely a Christian belief. Most religions assume people are born holy but may require forgiveness for sins they have perpetrated on earth (personal communication, Dr. John Lanci, February 18, 2001).

5. *Educate yourself concerning your client's religious beliefs.* Helpers should know about the religious affiliation of clients. They can learn by taking a course or workshop, by reading, by attending a client's place of worship, and if appropriate, by asking the client.

6. *Be familiar with holidays and traditions of your clients' religions.* So that helpers will not accidentally embarrass or offend their clients, they should become

familiar with the more important holidays and traditions of their clients' religion (e.g., a Muslim would not want to be offered food during the month of Ramadan).

7. *Understand that religion can deeply affect a client on many levels, including unconscious ones.* Some clients who deny any religious affiliation (e.g., "lapsed Catholics") may still be unconsciously driven by the basic values they were originally taught. Look at clients' actions; don't just listen to their words. For instance, a "lapsed Catholic" may continue to feel guilty over certain issues related to the religious beliefs he or she was taught.

8. *Know yourself.* Helpers should assess their own biases and prejudices to assure they will not negatively affect the helping relationship. Assessing any negative or positive feelings a helper may have toward any religious affiliation, including his or her own, will help assure that these feelings do not interfere with the helping relationship.

9. *Know appropriate skills.* Helpers should take courses and workshops and keep up with the most recent professional publications to assure that they know the most appropriate helping skills to use and *not use* with their clients.

Counseling Women

Because some mental health professionals were concerned with the ways that women were treated by helpers, the APA developed 13 guiding principles for helpers when working with women (Fitzgerald & Nutt, 1995) (see Box 9.2).

Believing that the guidelines did not go far enough, some have offered a more radical approach to working with women. These individuals believe that issues brought by women to helping relationships are inextricably related to oppression against women in society (Fitzgerald & Nutt, 1995; Gladding, 1996). They suggest that the helping relationship offers women an opportunity to develop their female identity and argue that female helpers can usually be most productive in this process (McNamara & Rickard, 1989). Downing and Roush (1985) offer one such model that includes five stages:

Stage I: Establish a relationship and demystify the helping relationship. Here helpers may downplay the "expert" role and encourage women to trust themselves. Helpers may identify with client issues and self-disclose as a way of forming a close relationship. They can assist in identifying social issues related to client problem(s) and use them to set goals.

Stage II: Validate and legitimize a woman's angry feelings toward her predicament. Here helpers assist clients to understand how they have been victimized through sociopolitical forces. Helpers assist clients in combating feelings of powerlessness, helplessness, and low self-esteem. They encourage participation in women's issues (reading books, attending seminars, taking part in women's groups).

BOX 9.2 Guidelines for Working with Women

1. Be aware of the biological, psychological, and social issues that impact women.
2. Be aware of how counseling theories and techniques help and/or hurt female clients.
3. Continually learn about special issues related to women and the helping relationship.
4. Recognize and be aware of all forms of oppression and how these interact with sexism.
5. Be knowledgeable of how verbal and nonverbal processes (particularly with regard to power in the relationship) affect women in the helping relationship.
6. Utilize skills that are particularly facilitative to women.
7. Do not have preconceived notions concerning the potential changes or goals of women.
8. Understand when it is best for a woman client to be seen by a female or male helper.
9. Use nonsexist language in counseling/therapy, supervision, teaching, and journal publication.
10. Do not engage in sexual activity with women clients under any circumstances.
11. Continually review your own values and biases and understand the effects of sex-role socialization upon your own development.
12. Be aware of how your personal functioning may influence the helping relationship with women clients. Monitor yourself through consultation, supervision, or your own therapy.
13. Support the elimination of sex bias within institutions and individuals.

(Adapted from Fitzgerald & Nutt, 1995, pp. 230–252)

Stage III: Provide a safe environment to express feelings as clients begin to form connections with other women. Here helpers validate feelings of fear and competition with other women that result from society's objectification of women. As these feelings dissipate, clients will move toward a strong and special connection to women. Helpers assist clients in understanding the difference between anger at a man and anger at a male-dominated system.

Stage IV: Help clients with conflicting feelings between traditional and newfound values. Here clients may feel torn between newfound feminist beliefs and values that do not seem congruent with those beliefs (e.g., wanting to stay home to raise the children). Helpers validate these contradictory feelings, acknowledge the confusion, and assist clients to fully explore their belief systems.

Stage V: Facilitate integration of client's new identity. Here helpers assist clients in integrating their newfound feminist beliefs with personal beliefs, even those personal beliefs that may not seem to be traditionally feminist. Clients are able to feel strength in their own identity development and no longer need to rely on an external belief system.

Counseling Men

You're not allowed to have issues; you're just a male.

(KRISTINA WILLIAMS-NEUKRUG)

When I was writing this section on men's issues in counseling, my wife said the above profound statement to me. You see, men in today's society are sometimes seen as not having issues because they have been in positions of power. And people in positions of power are often seen as holding a certain amount of privilege—which they do. However, helpers must be aware that there are men's issues and understand how such issues affect the helping relationship (Kelly & Hall, 1992; Osherson, 1986). A number of authors have offered ideas that can be incorporated into a set of guidelines when working with male clients (Osherson, 1986; Scher, 1981).

1. *Accept men where they are.* Men are particularly on guard when initially entering the helping relationship. Thus, the helper must accept men as they are in an effort to build trust. Once men feel safe, they work hard on their issues (Moore & Haverkamp, 1989; Scher, 1979).

2. *Don't push men to express what may be considered "softer feelings."* Men tend to be uncomfortable with the expression of certain feelings (e.g., deep sadness, feelings of incompetence, feelings of inadequacy, feelings of closeness) and more at ease with "thinking things through," problem solving, goal setting, and the expression of some other feelings, such as anger and pride. Push a man too quickly and he'll be pushed out of the helping relationship.

3. *Early on in therapy, validate the man's feelings.* To protect their egos, men tend to blame someone initially, often through anger at others and society, for their problems. Men need to feel validated in these feelings if they are to continue in the helping relationship.

4. *Validate the man's view of how he has been constrained by male sex-role stereotypes.* Early on in the helping relationship, note how the man is constrained by sex-role stereotypes and pressure in society (e.g., he must work particularly hard for his family). Validation of these views help to build trust and establish the relationship.

5. *Have a plan for therapy.* Men like structure and a sense of goal directedness—even if it is changed later on. Thus, the helper needs to be clear with men that he or she wants to collaborate with them on a plan for the helping relationship.

6. *Begin to discuss developmental issues.* Although each man has his own unique issues, he will likely also be struggling with common male developmental issues. The helper should be aware of and willing to discuss these issues (e.g., mid-life crises) (Levinson, 1986).

7. *Slowly encourage the expression of new feelings.* As trust is formed, men will begin to express what are typically considered more feminine feelings (e.g., tears, caring, feelings of intimacy). The helper should reinforce the expression of these newfound feelings.

8. *Explore underlying issues and reinforce new ways of understanding the world.* Expression of new feelings will lead to the emergence of underlying issues (e.g., childhood issues, feelings of inadequacy). One critical and painful issue for men is their relationship with their fathers. How fathers modeled, distanced themselves, and showed love becomes a template for men's relationships. The helper must help the male client "*heal his wounded father*" (Osherson, 1986).

9. *Explore behavioral change.* As men gain new insights into self, they may wish to try new ways of acting in the world. The client, in collaboration with the helper, can identify new potential behaviors and "try them out."

10. *Encourage the integration of newfound feelings, new ways of thinking about the world, and new behaviors into the man's lifestyle.* The expression of new feelings, newly gained insights, and new ways of thinking and acting will slowly take on a life of their own and be integrated into the client's way of living. Helpers can actively reinforce these new ways of being.

11. *Encourage new male relationships.* As male clients grow, new male friendships should be encouraged—friendships that allow the man to freely express his feelings while maintaining his "maleness." Men's groups can allow men to develop more intimate relationships with other men, feel supported, and be challenged to change (Moore & Haverkamp, 1989; Williams & Myer, 1992).

12. *Say goodbye.* Although some men may want to continue in the helping relationship, many will see it as time limited, a means to a goal. Thus, the helper should be able to say goodbye and end the relationship. Doing this sets the groundwork for the client to come back, if he so desires.

Counseling Gay Men and Lesbians

Although helpers should follow the general guidelines just discussed for counseling women and men when working with gays and lesbians, they should also remember that homosexuals have some unique concerns of their own. Thus, some authors have developed general guidelines for counseling gays and lesbians (Browning, Reynolds, & Dworkin, 1995; Pope, 1995; Shannon & Woods, 1995):

1. *Adopt a nonhomophobic attitude.* The helper should make sure that his or her biases do not interfere with the helping relationship.

2. *Make few assumptions about lifestyle.* Don't assume that a gay or lesbian client is comfortable living in what the dominant culture understands as

the gay and lesbian lifestyle. This lifestyle, which is often portrayed in movies and on TV, in fact is usually found only in larger metropolitan areas. The majority of lesbian and gay people in the United States inhabit a wide variety of "lifestyles."

3. *Know the unique issues of lesbians and gays.* By reading professional literature, and gay and lesbian literature, and by becoming involved with local lesbian and gay community groups, helpers can gain an understanding of some of the unique issues of gays and lesbians.

4. *Know community resources.* Be aware of community resources that might be useful to gays and lesbians.

5. *Know identity issues.* Be familiar with the identity development of gays and lesbians, especially as it relates to the coming out process (e.g., see Cass, 1979).

6. *Understand the idiosyncracies of religion toward homosexuality.* Be familiar with particular religions and spiritual concerns unique to lesbians and gays (e.g., some religions view homosexuality as abnormal).

7. *Be tuned into domestic violence issues.* Be aware that domestic violence can occur in gay and lesbian relationships just as it occurs in heterosexual relationships.

8. *Know about substance abuse.* Have a firm foundation in substance abuse treatment as gays and lesbians may have a greater tendency to misuse illegal substances as a method of dealing with the coming out process and the inherent prejudices in society (Dyne, 1990).

9. *Be knowledgeable about AIDS.* Although AIDS is not only a "gay disease," a disproportionate number of gay men are HIV positive and have AIDS.

10. *Know about sexual abuse.* Be particularly cognizant that a large percentage of lesbian women have been sexually abused before the age of 18 (38% according to Loulan, 1987).

Counseling Individuals Who Are HIV Positive

A number of challenges face the helper working with an individual who is HIV positive or who has AIDS. Shannon and Woods (1995) and others have highlighted some points to consider when counseling the individual with HIV:

1. *Know the cultural background of client.* HIV positive individuals are found in all cultural groups. In addition to dealing with issues unique to the HIV positive client, helpers may need to work on cross-cultural issues if the client is from a minority background.

2. *Know about the disease and combat myths.* Individuals who are HIV positive are discriminated against and feared. Helpers need to have knowledge about the disease so they will not be fearful and will be able to assist clients effectively when they are discriminated against.

3. *Be prepared to take on numerous helper roles.* When working with an individual who is HIV positive, a helper may need to be an advocate, counselor, caretaker, and resource person, or any of a number of other roles.

4. *Be prepared to deal with a number of unique treatment issues:*
   a. feelings about the loss of income due to the client's inability to work and/or the high cost of medical treatment
   b. depression and feelings of hopelessness concerning declining or uncertain health, and changes in the client's relationship to others
   c. the probability that the client will have friends and loved ones who are HIV positive or have died of AIDS if he or she is from a high-risk group

5. *Deal with your own feelings about mortality.* Finally, helpers will need to be able to deal effectively with their feelings about the client's possible impending death and how those feelings may bring to the surface issues concerning the helper's own immortality.

Counseling the Homeless and the Poor

A number of unique points should be considered when counseling the homeless and the poor (Axelson & Dail, 1988; Blasi, 1990; Rossi, 1990). Some of these include the following:

1. *Focus on social issues.* When working with individuals who are struggling with basic needs, it is important for the helper to focus on social issues, such as helping a person obtain food and housing, as opposed to working on intrapsychic issues.

2. *Know the racial/ethnic/cultural background of the client.* Because a disproportionate number of homeless and poor people come from nonmajority racial/ethnic/cultural groups, helpers will need to educate themselves about the cultural heritage of their clients.

3. *Be knowledgeable about health risks.* The homeless and the poor are at greater risk of developing AIDS, tuberculosis, and other diseases. The helper should have basic knowledge of such diseases, be able to do a basic medical screening, and have referral sources available.

4. *Be prepared to deal with multiple issues.* Because as many as 50% of the homeless are struggling with mental illness and/or substance abuse, helpers must often deal with the multiple issues of homelessness, poverty, mental illness, and chemical dependence.

5. *Know about developmental delays and be prepared to refer.* Homeless and poor children are more likely to have retarded language and social skills, be abused, and have delayed motor development; helpers should know how to identify developmental delays.

6. *Know psychological effects.* Helpers should know how to respond to clients' psychological and emotional reactions to homelessness and poverty, these can include despair, depression, and a sense of hopelessness (Blasi, 1990).

7. *Know resources.* Helpers should be aware of the vast number of resources available in the community and make referrals when appropriate.

Counseling Older Persons

Older persons present a different set of issues from younger people when they are counseled (Gibson & Mitchell, 1995; Schlossberg, 1995). To ensure that their concerns are addressed, helpers should consider the following:

1. *Adapt your counseling style.* The helper may need to adapt the helping relationship to fit the older client's needs. For instance, use journal writing or art therapy for older persons who have difficulty hearing. For nonambulatory clients, have a session in the client's home.

2. *Build a trusting relationship.* Older persons seek counseling at lower rates than other clients (Hashimi, 1991), and those who do may be less trustful, having been raised during a time when counseling was much less common. Helpers may need to spend additional time building a trusting relationship.

3. *Know potential sources of depression.* Depression can have many origins for the older person, including the loss of loved ones, lifestyle changes, and health issues. Helpers should be capable of identifying the many potential sources of depression.

4. *Know about identity issues.* Many older persons based their identities on their career, family, or roles in the community. These individuals may need to define themselves in new ways as they no longer function in their previous roles. Helpers can assist clients in finding a new sense of who they are.

5. *Be prepared to deal with feelings that result from changes in status.* Many older persons attained status through their life roles (e.g., in their careers, as the head of the house). Changes in these roles can lead to feelings of depression, anxiety, or despair.

6. *Know about possible and probable health changes.* Predictable changes in health can lead to depression and concern for the future. Unpredictable changes can lead to loss of income and emotional problems. Helpers should be alert to potential physical health problems and their emotional counterpart in the elderly.

7. *Have empathy for changes in interpersonal relationships.* Aging brings changes in significant relationships as a result of such things as the death of a spouse, partners, and friends; changes in health status; and relocation. Helpers should know about and have empathy toward their clients concerning these changes.

8. *Know about physical and psychological causes of sexual dysfunction.* Helpers should be aware of the possible physical and psychological causes of sexual dysfunction in the elderly. Helpers should also remember that regardless of age, people are always sexual beings.

Counseling People with Mental Illness

Helpers who work with the chronically mentally ill need to understand psychiatric disorders, psychotropic medications, and the unique needs of the chronically mentally ill such as homelessness, continual transitions, difficulty with employment, and dependent family relationships. Specific steps the helper can take when working with this population include the following:

1. *Helping the client understand his or her mental illness.* Many clients do not have an understanding of their illness, the usual course of the illness, and the best methods of treatment. Clients should be fully informed with up-to-date knowledge about their mental illness.

2. *Helping the client work through feelings concerning his or her mental illness.* Mental illness continues to be stigmatized in this society and many clients are embarrassed about their disorder. Support groups and a nonjudgmental attitude can help to normalize clients' views of themselves.

3. *Helping to assure attendance in counseling.* Clients may miss appointments because they are in denial about their illness, embarrassed, or simply do not care. Helpers can call clients the day before their appointment, have a relative or close friend help the client get to the helper's office, or work on specific strategies to help clients remember to come in for their appointments.

4. *Assuring compliance with medication.* Clients may discontinue medication out of forgetfulness, out of denial about the illness, because they believe they won't have a relapse, or because they believe medication is not helpful. Helpers need to be sure that clients continue to take their medication.

5. *Assuring accurate diagnosis.* Accurate diagnosis is crucial for treatment planning and the appropriate use of medication. Helpers can assure accurate diagnosis through testing, clinical interviews, interviews with others close to the client, and through appropriate use of supervision.

6. *Reevaluating the client's treatment plan and not giving up.* The mentally ill are some of the most difficult clients to work with and it is easy for helpers to become discouraged. Helpers need to continue to be vigilant about their work with the mentally ill and continually reevaluate treatment plans.

7. *Involving the client's family.* Some families can offer great support to clients, and they can be a window into the client's psyche. Thus, it is important to assure adequate family involvement and to help families understand the implications of the client's diagnosis.

8. *Knowing resources.* The mentally ill are often involved with many other resources in the community (e.g., Social Security disability, housing authority, support groups). It is therefore crucial that the helper have a working knowledge of these resources.

Counseling Individuals with Disabilities

As federal laws have increasingly supported the rights to services for individuals with disabilities, the helper has taken a more active role in their treatment and rehabilitation (Lombana, 1989). Observing the following treatment issues can help counselors provide positive services for this group.

1. *Have knowledge of the many disabling conditions.* Obviously, a helper cannot adequately work with an individual who has a disability if he or she does not understand the emotional and physical consequences of that disability.

2. *Help the client know his or her disability.* Clients should be fully informed of their disability, the probable course of treatment, and their prognosis. Knowledge of their disability will allow them to be fully involved in any emotional healing that needs to take place.

3. *Assist the client through the grieving process.* Clients who become disabled go through stages as they grieve their loss and accept their condition. Similar to people going through Kubler-Ross's (1997) stages of bereavement, clients can be expected to experience denial, anger, negotiation, resignation, and acceptance. The helper can facilitate the client's progress through these stages.

4. *Know referral resources.* Individuals with disabilities often have many needs. Thus, it is important that helpers are aware of community resources (e.g., physicians, social services, physical therapists, experts on pain management, vocational rehabilitation).

5. *Know the law and inform clients of the law.* By knowing the law the helper can assure that the client is receiving all necessary services and not being discriminated against. Helping clients understand the law empowers them by giving them the ability to protect their rights.

6. *Be prepared to do or refer clients for vocational/career counseling.* When faced with a disability, many people are also faced with making a career transition. Helpers should be ready either to do career/vocational counseling or refer a client to a career/vocational helper.

7. *Include the family.* Families can offer support, assist in long-term treatment planning, and help with the emotional needs of the client. Whenever reasonable, include the family.

8. *Be an advocate.* Individuals with disabilities are faced with prejudice and discrimination. Helpers can be client advocates by knowing the law, fighting for client rights, and assisting the client in fighting for his or her rights. A client who knows his or her rights and who acts as an advocate for himself or herself will feel empowered.

Exercise 9.4 gives you practice in interviewing clients from special populations.

EXERCISE 9.4   Attitudes, Knowledge, and Skills Needed for Special Populations

Interview an individual in one or more of the special populations listed below and ask the accompanying questions (and any other questions you think would be appropriate). Then, consider in small groups what attitudes, knowledge, and skills you would need to work with an individual from the particular group.

A. An Individual Who Has a Disability
1. How did you become disabled?
2. What unique experiences have you had related to your disability?
3. What prejudices have you experienced?
4. What social services have you used?
5. What social services would you like to have available?
6. Is there anything you would like to have changed about your life related to your current status?

B. An Individual Who Is Poor and/or Homeless
1. How did you become homeless or poor?
2. What unique experiences have you had related to your current life situation?
3. What prejudices have you experienced?
4. What social services have you used?
5. What social services would you like to have available?
6. How do you make it financially day-to-day?
7. What financial resources are available to you?

C. An Individual Who Is Gay or Lesbian
1. When did you discover you were gay or lesbian?
2. What internal "psychological" struggles did you have relative to your sexuality?
3. What unique experiences have you had related to your sexuality?
4. What prejudices have you experienced?
5. What social services, if any, have you used?
6. What social services, if any, would you like to have available?
7. Do you have any other thoughts related to society's attitude toward gays and lesbians?

D. An Individual Who Is HIV Positive
1. How did you become HIV positive?
2. What unique experiences have you had related to being HIV positive?
3. What prejudices have you experienced?
4. What social services have you used?
5. What social services would you like to have available?
6. What changes would you like to see take place in society related to your HIV positive status?

E. An Older Person
1. How do you feel about being an older person?
2. What unique experiences have you had related to your age?
3. What prejudices have you experienced?
4. What social services have you used?
5. What social services would you like to have available?
6. What attitudes related to aging would you like to see changed in society?

(Continued)

EXERCISE 9.4 Continued

F. An Individual Who Struggles with Mental Illness

1. When do you first remember having to deal with your mental health problems?
2. What unique experiences have you had related to your mental illness?
3. What prejudices have you experienced?
4. What social services have you used?
5. What social services would you like to have available?
6. Has medication assisted you with your mental health problems?
7. What changes in the mental health care delivery system would you like to see?

THE ETHICALLY ASTUTE CROSS-CULTURAL HELPER: ALWAYS CHANGING

The culturally different client deserves a human service professional who has left his or her biases behind, is knowledgeable about cultural and ethnic differences, and sensitive to the needs of the client (Cayleff, 1986; Quintana & Bernal, 1995). It is not surprising that our ethical guidelines speak to the importance of the following:

> Human service professionals should be knowledgeable of different cultures, be aware of their own cultural heritage and how that impacts others, understand sociopolitical issues, and be open to seeking ongoing training and supervision to work effectively with the culturally different client (see Statements 18, 19, 20, and 21, *Ethical Standards of Human Services Professionals,* see Appendix B)

As the ethical standards state, the effective human service professional who is cross-culturally astute is willing to examine his or her own cultural background. This individual understands that cultural awareness is developmental; that is, there are predictable stages through which we all will pass. We can understand the predictable stages through which we pass. Thus, we can gain an understanding of the typical behaviors we and others will exhibit as we pass through the stages. D'Andrea (1996) and D'Andrea and Daniels (1991) suggest that these stages range from an affective/impulsive stage of racism, in which a student may respond impulsively and in a hostile fashion to individuals from different backgrounds, to the principled activist stage in which students can understand and accept the reality that culturally different people may hold varying values and beliefs, and may behave in ways different from the helper. In addition, students in this final stage actively work for systemic change in society.

Helpers must continue to find the newest and best ways to assist all individuals with their emotional needs (Locke, 1992). Helpers must continue to examine new treatment approaches, explore new counseling theories, and be open to an expansive view of counseling for all individuals. As Romano (1992) wisely noted, "Not ours, not theirs; no one way of counseling surpasses another. . . . As cultures differ, so must counseling" (Romano, 1992, p. 1).

SUMMARY

In this chapter, we examined the reasons that knowledge of multicultural counseling is important in today's world. The face of America is rapidly changing, with minorities becoming an increasingly larger share of the population. Even so, minorities drop out of counseling at higher rates and are misdiagnosed more frequently than white clients.

Nine reasons to explain why the helping relationship does not seem to be working for minorities were explored: (1) Many helpers still believe in the melting pot myth; (2) clients and helpers often have incongruent expectations about the helping relationship; (3) some helpers lack understanding of the impact of social forces on minorities; (4) some helpers have an ethnocentric worldview; (5) most helpers are ignorant, at least to some degree, of their own racist attitudes and prejudices; (6) many helpers do not understand cultural differences in the expression of symptomatology; (7) helpers have to work with assessment and research instruments that are not as reliable with minorities as they are with white clients; (8) helpers often have to work with institutions (e.g., human service organizations) that continue to be inherently racist and inadequate when dealing with the counseling needs of minorities; and (9) the helping process has not been developed for clients from diverse backgrounds.

The chapter continued with an existential model for understanding the culturally different client. Helpers should attempt to understand the individual uniqueness of the client (eigenwelt), the common experiences that clients share with their cultural group (mitwelt), and shared universal experiences common to all clients (umwelt). Helpers should have appropriate beliefs and attitudes in that they should be aware of their own cultural backgrounds, biases, stereotypes, and values. They need to have knowledge of different ethnic and cultural groups, and possess specific skills necessary to work with culturally diverse clients.

A large portion of the chapter examined specific points to consider when working with a wide range of clients; individuals from ethnic and racial groups and from diverse religious backgrounds, women, men, gays and lesbians, those who are HIV positive, the homeless and the poor, older persons, the mentally ill, and individuals with disabilities. Finally, the astute cross-cultural helper is always changing in that he or she is always willing to examine himself or herself, and always willing to look at new ways to work with culturally different clients.

INFOTRAC COLLEGE EDITION

1. Search keyword "multicultural counseling" and research an aspect of your choice in more detail.

2. Research any of the specific groups listed in this chapter in more detail.

3. Research, in more detail, minority groups other than the ones listed in this chapter.

10

Ethical and Professional Issues

INTRODUCTION

This chapter presents an overview of some of the more prevalent ethical and professional issues related to the helping relationship, beginning with the purpose of ethical guidelines as well as some of their limitations. Next, the ethical decision-making process is reviewed along with some of the more prominent models now used and the impact of helpers' cognitive and moral development on the way they make ethical decisions. The remainder of the chapter examines some of the more important ethical and professional issues that human service professionals face, using ethical vignettes associated with these issues.

PURPOSE OF ETHICAL GUIDELINES

The National Organization for Human Service Education (NOHSE), in collaboration with the Council for Standards in Human Service Education (CSHSE), has always supported the concept of a code of ethics (Linzer, 1990), and in 1995 adopted its *Ethical Standards of Human Service Professionals* (see Appendix B). Although these guidelines have much in common with other codes of ethics (see ACA, 1995; APA, 1992; NASW, 1996), they also reflect the unique perspective and job requirements of the human service professional.

In the development of ethical standards, professional associations have wrestled with which societal and professional values the guidelines should reflect (see Neukrug, 1996; Neukrug, Lovell, & Parker, 1996). Ultimately, many of the mental health professional associations have developed ethical guidelines that share similar values and purposes (Ansell, 1984; Corey, Corey, & Callanan, 1998; Loewenberg & Dolgoff, 1996; Mabe & Rollin, 1986; Van-Zandt, 1990). Ethical codes have several purposes:

1. To protect consumers.
2. To further the professional stance of the organization.
3. To show that a profession has a particular body of knowledge and skills.
4. To assert the identity and provide an indication of the maturity of a profession.
5. To reflect underlying values of a profession and the behaviors that should follow those values.
6. To offer a framework for the ethical and professional decision-making process.
7. In case of litigation, to offer a defense for those who practice in accordance with the code.

Although ethical guidelines can assist practitioners in the ethical and professional decision-making process, they do have limitations (Mabe & Rollin, 1986):

1. Some issues cannot be handled in the context of a code.
2. There are some difficulties with enforcing the code.
3. It is often difficult to bring the client systematically into the code-construction process.
4. Issues in the code may be addressed by other methods, with results sometimes at odds with the code (for example, in the courts).
5. There are possible conflicts within a code or between two codes, the practitioner's values and the code, the code and ordinary morality, and the code and institutional practice.
6. Codes cannot cover all issues, especially new issues that arise.

Ethical guidelines are moral, *not legal,* documents, and our professional associations expect us to be bound by them. Sometimes, when a person violates the codes of ethics, he or she will be dismissed from the professional association. In some instances, states have incorporated part or all of a code of ethics into a legal document. In these cases, stiffer penalties such as fines or even imprisonment could result from an ethical violation.

ETHICAL DECISION MAKING: A COMPLEX PROCESS

Although the use of ethical guidelines is crucial when dealing with ethical dilemmas, good ethical decision making should be based on more than the sole use of these codes (Cottone & Tarvydas, 1998; Neukrug, 1996). As an aid in decision making, Corey, Corey, and Callanan (1998) developed a practical, problem-solving model that has eight steps: (1) identifying the problem, (2) identifying the potential issues involved, (3) reviewing the relevant ethical guidelines, (4) knowing relevant laws and regulations, (5) obtaining consultation, (6) considering possible and probable courses of action, (7) listing the consequences of various decisions, and (8) deciding on what appears to be the best course of action.

While the Corey model emphasizes the pragmatic aspects of ethical decision making, other theorists stress the role of moral principles in this process. For instance, Kitchener (1984) describes the role of five moral principles in the making of ethical decisions. In her view, mental health professionals should promote the autonomy of the client (e.g., self-determination, freedom of choice), should protect the good of others, should avoid causing harm to others, should seek justice and fairness for all, and should be committed to the helping relationship.

Some now suggest that ethical decision making may be influenced by the helper's level of ethical, moral, and cognitive development (Neukrug, 1996). Those who are at the lower developmental levels will view ethical decision making as a "black and white" or "right or wrong" process. Such human service professionals may rigidly rely on the ethical guidelines when making ethical decisions and might suggest there is a "correct" answer to an ethical dilemma. However, those at higher developmental levels would view ethical decision making as a more complex process. They will examine the ethical guidelines, will likely use a decision-making model such as that of Corey et al. and/or a moral model such as Kitchener's, and view the ethical decision-making process as a deep, self-reflective, and difficult process.

For instance, let's examine two human service professionals: Jason, who is at a lower developmental level, and Jawanda who is at a higher level. Both are faced with the same dilemma: A client of theirs is smoking crack cocaine and the agency at which they work requires that such individuals be reported to the administration who will then contact the police. Jason examines the ethical guidelines, reads the agency policy guidelines, and decides that the "right thing to do"—and the only choice he has—is to report his client to an administrator. Jawanda, however, views ethical decision making differently. She also reads the agency policy and reviews the ethical guidelines. In addition, she is likely to use a model such as that of Corey et al. or Kitchener in helping her decide what to do. She consults with others to gain other points of view, and only then carefully deliberates about what would be best for her client, the agency, society, and herself. After careful deliberation, she comes to a conclusion.

BOX 10.1   Becky

Reflect on the following vignette and then share your thoughts in small groups or with the class.

As a human service professional for the local department of human services, you have been assisting Becky, a single mother of a four-year-old daughter, for the past few years as she attempted to remove herself from the welfare rolls, obtain employment, and secure child care. Today, Becky walks into your office and tells you that she has been HIV-positive for the past eight years and that two years ago she developed AIDS. She has not responded well to her recent new regime of medication. She is clearly despondent, is very concerned for the well-being of her child, and confides to you that she is considering killing herself. She notes that she has few significant people in her life, realizes that it may only be a matter of time before she dies, and is concerned that in the time she has left she will not be able to adequately care for her daughter. She therefore would like your help in finding a good home for her child and in "getting her affairs in order" before she commits suicide. You are one of her few confidantes, and she is someone you care about. As a helper, what should you do?

The conclusion in this case is really less important than the process, as Jawanda has dealt with the situation in a complex and thoughtful manner as opposed to Jason's somewhat hasty decision making. In fact, although both may come to the same conclusion, I would rather work with someone like Jawanda because she shows thoughtfulness and the ability to self-reflect—qualities I would want in a colleague (and a friend!). Thus, one can see that ethical decision making can and perhaps should be a complex process. As you review the ethical dilemma presented in Box 10.1, use the ethical guidelines, a model such as that of Corey et al. or Kitchener, consult with others, and consider what is best for the client, the agency, the human service professional, and society when making your decision.

SELECTED ETHICAL ISSUES
AND ETHICAL DILEMMAS

Following are descriptions of some of the more prevalent ethical issues faced today by human service professionals. These issues are followed by ethical vignettes related to those issues. In reviewing these issues and responding to the vignettes, consider the points made earlier in the chapter and refer to the *Ethical Standards of Human Service Professionals,* Appendix B.

Informed Consent

Already discussed in Chapter 6, informed consent involves the client's right to know the purpose and nature of all aspects of client involvement with the helper and within the helping relationship. Today, an increasing number of writers in the field are recommending that clients sign informed-consent forms indicating that they are fully aware of any procedures in which they are participating (Bray, Shepherd, & Hays, 1985; Handelsman, Kemper, Kesson-Craig, McLain, & Johnsrud, 1986). Often, such informed consent is given after a mental health professional has furnished the client with a professional disclosure statement that explains issues such as these:

1. the limits of confidentiality
2. the purpose of the interview
3. the limits of the relationship
4. legal concerns of helper and client
5. agency rules that might affect the client
6. the length of the interview
7. the helper's credentials
8. the theoretical orientation of the helper
9. fees for services
10. any other relevant information

Obtaining informed consent from a client used to be something that was given lip service. Today, however, ethical guidelines highlight the importance to all human service professionals of having this consent:

> Human service professionals negotiate with clients the purpose, goals, and nature of the helping relationships prior to its onset, as well as inform clients of the limitations of the proposed relationship. (Statement 1, *Ethical Standards of Human Service Professionals,* see Appendix B.)

Ethical Vignettes Related to Informed Consent

1. You decide to refer a client because you have not worked with a situation like hers before and feel that it's out of your area of expertise. She becomes livid, stating that you did not warn her of this possibility in your informed consent statement. Does she have a point? Can everything be explained in an informed consent statement?

2. A human service professional gives a written document to a family explaining the limitations to confidentiality and the general direction the family sessions will take. After reading this *informed consent document,* the parents sign it and bring in the family. The informed consent document is not given to or described to the children. Has the helper acted ethically? Professionally?

3. In the course of a conversation with a client, you discover that she has been smoking marijuana. An agency rule is that any client suspected of using illegal drugs must be immediately referred to rehabilitation, and if he or she refuses, you can no longer see the client at your agency. You explain this to her, she gets angry, walks out, and says she's going to sue because you did not previously explain this to her. Does she have a point?

Competence and Scope of Knowledge

Helper competence is consistently acknowledged as a crucial ethical concern by most professional associations (Corey, Corey, & Callanan, 1998). Knowing one's level of competence and having the desire to learn new skills that would be effective with a broad range of clients is essential for the human service professional (Frank, 1979; Kanfer & Goldstein, 1991; Lacrosse, 1980). Knowing the limits of one's professional knowledge is also important:

> Human service workers know the limit and scope of their professional knowledge and offer services only within their knowledge and skill base. (Statement 26, *Ethical Standards of Human Service Professionals*, see Appendix B.)

> Human service professionals continually seek out new and effective approaches to enhance their professional abilities. (Statement 31, *Ethical Standards of Human Service Professionals*, see Appendix B.)

In an effort be as effective as possible with clients, helpers must continually seek out new professional opportunities to enhance their work. In fact, it is unethical *not* to seek out such activities:

> Human service workers promote the continuing development of their profession. They encourage membership in professional associations, support research endeavors, foster educational advancement, advocate appropriate legislative actions, and participate in other related professional activities. (Statement 30, *Ethical Standards of Human Service Professionals*, see Appendix B.)

Ethical Vignettes Related to Competence and Scope of Practice

1. A human service professional attends a number of workshops in Gestalt therapy, an advanced therapeutic approach. He feels assured about his skills and decides to run a Gestalt therapy group. The state in which he works licenses counselors, psychologists, and social workers as therapists, but not human service professionals. Is it ethical and legal for him to run such a group?

2. A human service worker with an associate-level (two-year) degree who is planning to return to school to obtain his bachelor's and master's degrees, tells his colleagues that he is a "master's degree candidate." Is this person misrepresenting himself? Might clients be confused by the term "master's degree candidate?" Is this ethical? Professional? Legal?

3. You are working with a client who begins to share bizarre thoughts concerning the end of the world. You decide that this individual needs special attention, so you spend extra time with him. Is this appropriate? Ethical? Professional? Legal?

4. A client tells a human service professional that she is taking Prozac, an antidepressant, and it isn't having any effect. She asks advice on increasing

the dosage and the human service professional states, "If the current dosage isn't working, consider taking a higher dosage." Is this response appropriate? Ethical? Professional? Legal?

5. A human service professional who has received specialized training in directing parenting workshops on communication skills decides to run a workshop at the local Holiday Inn. She rents a room and runs an ad in the local newspaper that reads "Learn How to Talk to Your Kid—Rid Your Family of All Communication Problems." Should she do the workshop? Is this ad ethical? Professional? Legal?

Supervision

One method of seeking out new and effective approaches to the helping relationship is through supervision. Supervision allows the helper to examine his or her view of human nature, theoretical approach, ability at implementing techniques, and, ultimately, his or her effectiveness with clients. Supervision should start during a helper's training program, "serve as a unique link between preparation and skilled service" (Cogan & O'Connell, 1982, p. 12), and continue as long as a person is working with clients in the human service field. There is nothing better than a good supervisory relationship that is based on trust, mutual respect, and understanding to assist helpers in taking a good look at what they are doing (Sadow, Ryder, Stein, & Geller, 1987).

The supervisor has a number of roles and responsibilities that include assuring the welfare of the client; making sure that ethical, legal, and professional standards are being upheld; overseeing the clinical and professional development of the supervisee; and evaluating the supervisee (ACES, 1995). It is the responsibility of the human service professional to seek out supervision when questions and concerns about the helping relationship arise.

> Human service professionals seek appropriate consultation and supervision to assist in decision-making when there are legal, ethical or other dilemmas. (Statement 27, *Ethical Standards of Human Service Professionals*, see Appendix B.)

Like the effective helper, the "good" supervisor is empathic, flexible, genuine, and open (Borders, 1994; Neukrug, 2000). In addition, the good supervisor is comfortable evaluating the supervisee and being an authority figure (Bradley & Gould, 1994). Good supervisors know and understand the helping relationship, have good client conceptualization skills, and are good problem solvers.

Unfortunately, all too often I have seen professionals avoid supervision because of fears about their own adequacy. These fears can create an atmosphere of isolation for the human service professional, an isolation that leads to rigidity and an inability to examine varying methods of working with clients. Professionals must face their vulnerable spots in an effort to examine what they do well and what they don't do well.

Ethical Vignettes Related to Supervision

1. A human service professional decides to pay lip service to her supervisor because she does not like him. She tells her co-workers that her supervisor is "stupid" and does not know what he's talking about. What, if anything, is unethical about this behavior? What should the human service professional do? What should her colleagues do?

2. Your supervisor tells you that he is going to have to report your client to social services for possible child abuse. You believe that he would be breaking the confidentiality of your relationship with your client. Is what he's doing ethical? Professional? Legal?

3. After meeting with a supervisee, the supervisor believes the supervisee's client is in danger of harming herself. The supervisee believes the client is not a risk and decides not to take action despite requests by the supervisor. The supervisor decides to contact the client herself and arranges to have her committed to a psychiatric unit. Has the supervisee acted ethically? Professionally? Has the supervisor acted ethically? Professionally?

4. In offering a professional disclosure statement to clients a helper fails to tell the clients that she is being supervised. Is this ethical? Professional?

5. A supervisor believes that a helper is doing harm to a client and insists the helper change his approach. The helper argues that he believes he is helping the client. The supervisor tells the helper either to change his approach or be fired. Has the supervisee acted ethically? Professionally? Has the supervisor acted ethically? Professionally?

6. A supervisee believes that her supervisor is incompetent and giving her poor supervision. She decides to report him to his superior. Has she acted ethically? Professionally? Is there anything else she could have done?

Confidentiality

Keeping client information confidential is one of the most important ingredients in building a trusting relationship. However, is confidentiality always guaranteed or warranted? For instance, suppose you encounter the following situation:

> A 17-year-old client tells you that she is pregnant. Do you need to tell her parents? What if the client was 15 or 12? What if she was drinking while pregnant, or using cocaine? What if she tells you she wants an abortion? What if she tells you she is suicidal because of the pregnancy?

Although most of us would agree that confidentiality is an important ingredient in the helping relationship, it may not always be the best course. All ethical decisions are to some degree a judgment call, but some general guidelines can be followed when you are making a decision to break confidentiality (always check local laws, however, to see if there are variations). Generally, confidentiality can be broken:

BOX 10.2   The Tarasoff Case

The case of *Tarasoff v. Board of Regents of University of California* (1976) set a precedent for the responsibility that mental health professionals have regarding maintaining confidentiality and acting to prevent a client from harming self or others. This case involved a client who was seeing a psychologist at the University of California at Berkeley health services. The client told the psychologist that he intended to kill Tatiana Tarasoff, his former girlfriend. After the psychologist consulted with his supervisor, the supervisor suggested that he call the campus police. Campus security subsequently questioned the client and released him. The client refused to see the psychologist any longer, and two months later he killed Tatiana. The parents of Tatiana sued and won, with the California Supreme Court stating that the psychologist did not do all that he could to protect Tatiana. Although state laws vary on how to handle confidentiality, this case generally is seen as signifying to mental health professionals they have a "duty-to-warn" individuals and must break confidentiality when the public's safety is at risk. Generally, they must do all that is reasonably possible to assure that a person is not harmed. In this case, contacting Tatiana Tarasoff may have been the prudent thing to do.

---

1. if a client is in danger of harming himself or herself or someone else (see Box 10.2). This is known as "duty-to-warn."

2. if a child is a minor and the law states that parents have a right to information about their child.

3. if a client asks the helper to break confidentiality (for example, your testimony is needed in court).

4. if a helper is bound by the law to break confidentiality (for example, a local law that requires human service professionals to report the selling of drugs).

5. to reveal information about a client to the helper's supervisor in order to benefit the client.

6. when a helper has a written agreement from his or her client to reveal information to specified sources (for example, other social service agencies that are working with the same client).

There are times when breaking confidentiality is not permissible. Generally, it is not appropriate when

1. the helper is frustrated with a client and he or she talks to a friend or colleague about the case just to "let off steam."

2. a helping professional requests information about his or her client and has not received written permission from the client to do so.

3. a friend asks a helper to tell him or her something interesting about a client with whom the helper is working.

4. breaking confidentiality will clearly cause harm to a client and does not fall into one of the categories listed earlier.

Not surprisingly, the *Ethical Standards of Human Service Professionals* (see Appendix B) reflects these statements and ensures the right to confidentiality, except when certain conditions exist.

Human service professionals protect the right to privacy and confidentiality except when such confidentiality would cause harm to the client or to others, when agency guidelines state otherwise, or under other stated conditions (e.g., local, state, or federal laws). Professionals inform clients of the limits of confidentiality prior to the onset of the relationship. (Statement 3, *Ethical Standards of Human Service Professionals,* see Appendix B.)

Ethical Vignettes Related to Confidentiality

1. After working at an agency for a few months, you realize that employees there are committing many breaches of confidentiality. What, if anything should you do?

2. After working at an agency for a few months, you realize that many of your co-workers tend to make fun of their clients during break. What, if anything should you do?

3. In your conversation with a client at the homeless shelter, you discover that he is drinking and taking Quaaludes in amounts that you believe could kill him. You mention this to him, but he tells you to mind your own business. What do you do?

4. In the course of working with a client, she expresses her concern about her grandmother who, she states, lives by herself, is depressed, has stopped eating, and has lost a considerable amount of weight. You contact the grandmother, but she refuses services. What do you do?

5. While you are talking with a 15-year-old male client, he informs you that on a recent vacation he was sexually molested by an uncle. He asks you not to tell his parents. What do you do?

6. A 15-year-old client tells you he is having sexual relations with his 14-year-old stepsister. What do you do?

7. A client of yours tells you that from time to time, usually when she's drinking, she gets severely depressed and thinks about killing herself. You ask her if she has a plan, and she says, "Well, sometimes I think about just doing it with that gun my husband has." One day she calls you; she's been drinking, and she tells you she's depressed. She hangs up saying "I don't know what I might do." What do you do?

8. While you are helping a client find preparation classes for the GED exam, she reveals that sometimes when she's drinking she takes the belt out and "whacks my kids good 'cause they just won't shut up." Do you break confidentiality and tell child protective services?

9. A client who is receiving services in your agency demands to see her case notes. In them, you have noted that you suspect she may be lying about her Social Security eligibility and that you also suspect she might be paranoid. What do you do?

10. A client you have been seeing at a crisis center comes in and asks to see all records pertaining to him. These include crisis logs that have information in them about other clients, as well as case notes you have made concerning his contacts. What do you do?

Privileged Communication

Generally, the confidentiality of written or oral communication between human service professionals and their clients is not protected under the law. This is because human service professionals do not have the legal protection afforded to licensed professionals under the legal term *privileged communication.* Whereas confidentiality is generally described in one's ethical standards and speaks to the importance of keeping client information in confidence, privileged communication is decreed by state legislatures and refers to information that can legally be held in confidence (Remember: Ethical guidelines are not legal documents!).

A recent ruling appears to uphold the right to confidentiality of records if one is a licensed professional who has privileged communication (*Jaffee v. Redmond,* 1996; see Box 10.3). In this case, the Supreme Court held the right of a licensed social worker to keep her case records confidential. Describing the social worker as a "therapist" and "psychotherapist," the ruling will likely protect all licensed social workers in federal courts and may protect all licensed therapists in all courts (Remley, Herlihy, & Herlihy, 1997). Although it's heartening that this case upheld the right to confidentiality of a licensed professional, it almost assuredly does not apply to the human service professional.

Ethical Vignettes Related to Privileged Communication

1. You a working with a women who is divorcing her husband. Suddenly, you receive a subpoena to go to court to discuss information about your client for a child custody battle the couple is having. You decide to go to court but do not reveal any information, stating, "This is confidential information; I refuse to reveal anything." Are you acting ethically? Legally?

2. A licensed social worker tells you that she was recently asked to reveal information about her client who was being sued for injuring a person while driving intoxicated. The social worker refused to reveal any information and was cited by the judge for contempt of court. The social worker is appealing the case stating she has privileged communication and does not have to reveal such information. Does she have a point? What if this was a human service professional?

3. A client's husband shows up at your office demanding information about his wife. You tell him things are confidential and privileged. He tells you

---

BOX 10.3   Jaffee v. Redmond

Mary Lu Redmond, a police officer in a village near Chicago, responded to a "fight in progress" call at an apartment complex on June 27, 1991. At the scene, she shot and killed a man she believed was about to stab another man he was chasing. The family of the man she had killed sued Redmond, the police department, and the village, alleging that Officer Redmond had used excessive force in violation of the deceased's civil rights. When the plaintiff's lawyers learned that Redmond had sought and received counseling from a licensed social worker employed by the village, they sought to compel the social worker to turn over her case notes and records and testify at the trial.

Redmond and the social worker claimed that their communications were privileged under an Illinois statute. They both refused to reveal the substance of their counseling sessions even though the trial judge rejected their argument that the communications were privileged. The judge then instructed jurors that they could assume that the information withheld would have been unfavorable to the policewoman, and the jury awarded the plaintiffs $545,000. (Remley, Herlihy, & Herlihy, 1997, p. 214)

After a series of appeals, the case was heard by the Supreme Court on February 26, 1996. The Court decided that the licensed therapist did indeed hold privileged communication and that the judge's instruction to the jury was therefore unwarranted.

---

that he'll sue you and the rest of this "flea bag" operation and that you do not hold privilege. Does he have a point?

4. Referring to item 3 above. Even though you do not hold privilege, must you share information about your client with the husband? If the husband came to you with a letter from his lawyer asking for such information, how would you respond?

Dual Relationships and the Human Service Worker

Is it all right to have as a client a friend, relative, or lover? Most professional groups have taken clear stands that this is not ethical. For instance, the *Ethical Standards of Human Service Professionals* (see Appendix B) strongly discourages dual relationships:

> Human service professionals are aware that in their relationship with clients, power and status are unequal. Therefore they recognize that dual or multiple relationships may increase the risk of harm to, or exploitation of, clients, and may impair their professional judgement. However, in some communities and situations it may not be feasible to avoid social or other nonprofessional contact with clients. Human service professionals support the trust implicit in the helping relationship by avoiding dual relationships that may impair professional judgment, increase risk of harm to clients or lead to exploitation. (Statement 6, *Ethical Standards of Human Service Professionals*, see Appendix B.)

Because human service professionals are not involved in intensive psychotherapeutic relationships, the relationship with their clients differs from those of counselors and psychologists. I believe, however, that it is the responsibility of each human service professional to decide whether his or her objectivity and professional judgment are impaired by having a dual relationship with a client. Generally, it is not wise to have a dual relationship; in almost every case, another human service worker can help that individual.

Ethical Vignettes Related to Dual Relationships

1. While driving to work one day, your car breaks down. A client of yours sees you and says "I'm good with mechanical things; let me help for a small fee. Besides I could use a little money for buying my motorcycle." You want to get your car fixed, and you want your client to have his bike. Do you let him help you?

2. For months you have been encouraging a client to get involved in more social activities. One day your client shows up at your art class saying that she signed up for the same class. What do you do?

3. You work for social services and are assigned to see Mr. Jones for Temporary Assistance for Needy Families (TANF) (welfare). As soon as Mr. Jones walks into your office, you realize that it is your neighbor from down the street. You don't know him that well and decide to meet with him. Is this ethical? Why or why not?

4. Using the vignette in number 3, when Mr. Jones walks in you realize he is your next-door neighbor, with whom you are fairly friendly. What do you do?

5. One of the secretaries in your office asks to see you "informally" to discuss a problem she is having with her child. After meeting with her for a few minutes, you realize that your "informal" meeting is becoming pretty "heavy" and "therapeutic." What do you do? Is this a dual relationship?

Sexual Relationships with Clients

A particular kind of dual relationship, sexual relationships with clients, has consistently been one of the most frequently lodged complaints made against mental health professionals (Neukrug, Milliken, & Walden, 2001). Because a sexual relationship with a client is among the most damaging of all ethical violations (Herlihy & Corey, 1997; Somer & Saadon, 1999), virtually all helping professions have issued prohibitions against it, and 15 states have made such actions a felony (Foster, 1996).

Sexual relationships with current clients are not considered to be in the best interest of the client and are prohibited. Sexual relationships with previous clients are considered dual relationships and are addressed in Statement 6. (Statement 7, *Ethical Standards of Human Service Professionals*, see Appendix B.)

Sexual relationships with clients can, and usually do, cause serious psychological harm to clients. Thus, human service professionals must understand the inherent problems with this kind of relationship, the legal implications this violation carries, and the ways in which helpers can manage their sexual feelings toward clients without acting on them (Herlihy & Corey, 1997; Pope & Tabachnick, 1993).

Ethical Vignettes Related to Sexual Relationships with Clients

1. You are becoming increasingly attracted to one of your clients, and even though you have no intention of acting on your feelings, you realize that you cannot concentrate as fully as you would like. Is this a dual relationship? What should you do?

2. Because you are becoming increasingly attracted to one of your clients, you decide to be honest with him and share your feelings. Is this appropriate? Why or why not?

3. You suspect that a colleague of yours is having a sexual relationship with one of his clients. What should you do?

4. You are working at a crisis center that has a number of volunteer workers. You become attracted to one of the volunteers, who used to be one of your clients but is no longer in treatment. You decide to have a relationship with her (him). Is this appropriate? Is this ethical?

Primary Obligation: Client, Agency, or Society?

Based on the *Ethical Standards of Human Service Professionals,* (see Appendix B) a client's right for self-determination and respect clearly should be honored by human service professionals.

The client's right to self-determination is protected by human service professionals. They recognize the client's right to receive or refuse services. (Statement 2, *Ethical Standards of Human Service Professionals,* see Appendix B.)

Human service professionals respect the integrity and welfare of the client at all times. Each client is treated with respect, acceptance and dignity. (Statement 8, *Ethical Standards of Human Service Professionals,* see Appendix B.)

Despite this emphasis in the ethical guidelines, there may be times when a client's right is superseded by other concerns. For instance, examine the scenario below.

In building your relationship with a 17-year-old client, you discover that she is taking the drug ecstasy, possibly selling drugs to friends, and involved in gang violence including looting. Your agency has a policy to report any illegal acts to the "proper authorities."

Does the client have the right to sell drugs, be involved in gang violence, and loot? What is your responsibility to this client? What are the limits of confidentiality with her? If you are primarily responsible to your client, what are the implications of your being required to report her to the proper authorities? If you do not report her to the proper authorities as you are supposed to do, what implications might this have on your employment? What responsibility do you have to protect society from the illegal activities in which she is involved? What liability concerns do you have if you do not report the illegal acts in which she is participating?

After examining the above scenario, you probably would agree that there may be times when a client's right to self-determination and respect is superseded by a helper's ethical obligation to protect others and to protect society. Along these lines, the *Ethical Standards of Human Service Professionals* (see Appendix B) suggests that the human service professional should seek out consultation and/or supervision and even break confidentiality if anyone is at risk of being harmed.

> If it is suspected that danger or harm may occur to the client or to others as a result of a client's behavior, the human service professional acts in an appropriate and professional manner to protect the safety of those individuals. This may involve seeking consultation, supervision, and/or breaking the confidentiality of the relationship. (Statement 4, *Ethical Standards of Human Service Professionals,* see Appendix B.)

The same standards also require that the human service worker follow agency guidelines, whenever reasonable, as well as local, state, and federal laws.

> Human service professionals protect the client's right to privacy and confidentiality except when such confidentiality would cause harm to the client or others, when agency guidelines state otherwise, or under other stated conditions (e.g., local, state, or federal laws). Professionals inform clients of the limits of confidentiality prior to the onset of the helping relationship. (Statement 3, *Ethical Standards of Human Service Professionals,* see Appendix B.)

Although clients generally have the right to confidentiality, the right to be respected, and the right for self-determination, human service professionals also recognize and sometimes favor the right of other individuals and of society in general to be protected from harm.

Ethical Vignettes Related to Obligation to Client, Agency, or Society

1. Your agency has implemented a new policy that all clients who are using illegal drugs will be reported to the police. You vigorously oppose such a policy and decide to ignore it. Are you acting ethically? Professionally? Legally?

2. An adult client informs you that he wants to kill his ex-girlfriend and her new boyfriend. He denies that he actually will act on these feelings but that he just "thinks about it a lot." What do you do?

3. You're working for social services, and in the course of a conversation with a client you discover that she has been using heroin. An agency dictate states that any client suspected of using illegal drugs must be immediately referred to rehabilitation, and if he or she refuses, you can no longer

see the client at your agency. You explain this to her, she gets angry, walks out, and states she'll "blow this place up." What do you do?

4. The director of the agency in which you work tells all employees to report any client who is using illegal substances to the police. Can the director do this? Is this ethical? Professional? What, if anything, should you do?

5. A client of yours, who has stopped taking his medication, stops by your office and seems pretty angry. He says, "That cheating Harley-Davidson dealer, he's trying to rip me off. He told me I could have that bike at discount and went back on his word." You try to talk with your client, but he storms out of your office saying "I'm going to get that man!" What do you do?

6. A married client of yours tells you she is pregnant by her neighbor. She's going to have an abortion. Your state has a law requiring women to tell their spouses if they're to have an abortion. She refuses. What do you do?

Continuing Education

Education never ends. Although you obtain a degree and work hard for it, to be effective throughout your career as a human service professional, you must never stop learning. Today, boards of registration, certification, and/or licensing are increasingly requiring continuing education for professionals to maintain their professional credentials. This requirement ensures that the professional is continuing to learn and that he or she can offer the best services possible to his or her clients. Continuing education is both our professional and ethical obligation:

> Human service professionals continually seek out new and effective approaches to enhance their professional abilities.

> [They] encourage membership in professional associations, support research endeavors, foster educational advancement, advocate for appropriate legislative actions, and participate in other related professional activities. (Statements 30 and 31, *Ethical Standards of Human Service Professionals,* see Appendix B.)

Once you are in the field, you will find that there are gaps in your education and discover that issues that were not stressed in your training now seem essential for you to know at work. Therefore, continuing education beyond your degree is essential. You can accomplish this through a variety of means including joining professional associations and participating in workshops they sponsor, participating in staff development workshops where you work, and taking additional coursework, perhaps to earn an advanced degree.

As you continue through your career, you will refine your skills, learn new ways of responding to clients, and become more grounded in your approach. It's like continually finding yourself—rediscovering your voice and making it clearer. Carl Rogers used to say that as an individual goes through his or her self-discovery process, choices become clearer—almost as if one does not have a choice because his or her path in life becomes obvious (Rogers, 1989). I believe a similar process occurs as we develop as professionals. Our skills, abilities, and who we are within the helping relationship become increasingly refined and more focused. It's as if we have little choice in how we should act within the relationship—we become the expert!

Ethical Vignettes Related to Continuing Education

1. After obtaining your first job you discover that many of your human service colleagues have forgotten the theories they once learned in school and do not feel obligated to engage in continuing education. What is your responsibility in this situation? What is your ethical obligation?

2. A colleague seems to have rigid views about his clients and refuses to participate in continuing education activities. He says, "I've been in this field a long time; I know what I'm doing." Is he acting ethically? Professionally? What, if anything should you do?

3. A colleague tells you that she is only working with female clients who have been abused. She encourages all her clients to leave their husbands and states that this is the "right thing to do" from a feminist perspective. Does she have a point? Is what she's doing ethical? Professional? Legal?

4. A human service professional of 20 years is your colleague. He does not belong to his professional associations. He never attends any continuing education workshops. He is not abreast of new information in the field. Is this ethical? Is this professional?

5. A human service professional you know has attended a number of workshops on substance abuse, obtained "certificates of attendance," and now advertises that he is certified in substance abuse counseling. Is this ethical? Professional? Legal? What, if anything, should you do?

Multicultural Counseling

The identity of mental health professionals has long been based on a Western/European model that tends to embrace the values and beliefs of white clients while negating the values and beliefs of minority clients. If counseling is to be an equal opportunity profession, helpers must graduate from training programs with more than a *desire* to help all people. As a profession, we will have achieved competence in working with diverse clients only when each graduate of a training program has learned helping strategies that can work for a wide range of clients, has worked with clients from diverse backgrounds, and leaves his or her program with an appreciation for diversity and an identity as a helper that includes a multicultural perspective (Essandoh, 1996).

Whitfield (1994) suggests that each mental health professional

1. be multilingual, in that they have obtained some working knowledge of the language of clients with whom they work,

2. have a multicultural view, in that they understand values and ways of living in the world of many different people,

3. is multiculturally literate, in that they know about important works of art and writings from other cultures,

4. is ethnically informed, in that they understand the unique customs and habits of people from various cultures,

5. and is ecologically literate, in that they have knowledge of the environment from which the client comes and how it affects their way of living in the world.

The *Ethical Standards of Human Service Professionals* supports this view. In a series of ethical statements, it notes that there is a necessity not to discriminate; it stresses the importance of having knowledge of the culture and communities within which the human service professional practices, the necessity of knowing one's own biases and stereotypes, the value of advocacy for minorities, and the importance of seeking the training, experience, education, and supervision necessary when working with minority clients (see statements 16 through 21 of the *Ethical Standards of Human Service Professionals,* see Appendix B).

Ethical Vignettes Related to Multicultural Counseling

1. Because of cross-cultural differences, you believe that your work with an Asian client has not been successful. Rather than referring the client, you decide to read more about your client's culture to gain a better understanding of him. Is this ethical? Is this professional?

2. You discover some fellow students making sexist jokes. What should you do? Have you encountered such behavior? Do you have any ethical, professional, and or moral responsibility in this situation?

3. You find some family members making ethnic/cultural slurs. What should you do? Have you encountered such behavior? Do you have any ethical, professional, and or moral responsibility in this situation?

4. A colleague of yours identifies herself as a feminist. You know that when she works with some women, she actively encourages them to leave their husbands when she discovers the husband is verbally or physically abusive. Is she acting ethically? Should you do anything?

5. You discover that a colleague of yours is telling a homosexual client that he is acting immorally. What should you do? Is this ethical? Professional? Legal?

6. A friend of yours advertises that she is a Christian counselor. You discover that when clients come to see her, she encourages them to read parts of the Bible during sessions and tells clients they need to ask for repentance for their sins. Is this ethical? Is this professional? Is this legal?

7. When working with an Asian client who is not expressive of her feelings, a helper you know pressures the client to express feelings. The helper tells the client, "You can only get better if you express yourself." Is this helper acting ethically? Professionally? Do you have any responsibility in this case?

8. When offering a parenting workshop to individuals who are poor, you are challenged by some of the parents when you tell them that "hitting a child is never okay." They tell you that you are crazy, and that sometimes a good spanking is the only thing that will get the child's attention. Do they have a point? How should you respond?

SUMMARY

This chapter reviewed important ethical and professional issues related to the helping relationship. An important element is ethical guidelines; these ethical codes (1) help to protect consumers, (2) further professionalism, (3) denote a body of knowledge for the profession, (4) assert the identity and maturity of a profession, (5) reflect a profession's underlying values and suggested behaviors, (6) offer a framework for making ethical decisions, and (7) can be used, in a court of law, as support for the professional if the professional acted appropriately.

Some limitations of ethical guidelines are that (1) some issues cannot be handled with a code, (2) there are some difficulties in enforcing codes, (3) the public is often not included in the code construction process, (4) issues addressed by codes are sometimes handled in other ways (e.g., the courts), (5) there are possible values and morals conflicts between a code and practitioners and between a code and society, and (6) codes cannot cover all issues.

Professionals can use models to help them make ethical decisions, such as the decision-making model by Corey et al. and the moral principle model of Kitchener. Dualists and relativists make ethical decisions differently, as the dualist tends see ethical decision making as black or white, while the relativist tends to make ethical decisions in a much more complex fashion.

The rest of the chapter focused on some of the more important ethical and professional issues that human service professionals face: informed consent, competence and scope of knowledge, supervision, the importance of confidentiality, privileged communication, dual relationships, primary obligation, continuing education, and multicultural counseling.

With all these issues, statements from the *Ethical Standards of Human Service Professionals* (see Appendix B) that addressed them were highlighted. In addition, ethical vignettes were offered to generate discussion about these important topics.

 INFOTRAC COLLEGE EDITION

1. Research the *"Jaffee v. Redmond"* decision and examine its impact on privileged communication for differing mental health professionals.

2. Examine the importance of "duty-to-warn" in various professions.

3. Choose any of the ethical issues presented in this chapter and research it in more detail.

Appendix A

Competency Areas
for Skills Standards

Competency 1: Participant Empowerment	The competent community support human service practitioner (CSHSP) enhances the ability of the participant to lead a self-determining life by providing the support and information necessary to build self-esteem, and assertiveness; and to make decisions. (p. 21)
Competency 2: Communication	The community support human service practitioner should be knowledgeable about the range of effective communication strategies and skills necessary to establish a collaborative relationship with the participant. (p. 26)
Competency 3: Assessment	The community support human service practitioner should be knowledgeable about formal and informal assessment practices in order to respond to the needs, desires and interests of the participants. (p. 29)
Competency 4: Community and Service Networking	The community support human service practitioner should be knowledgeable about the formal and informal supports available in his or her community and skilled in assisting the participant to identify and gain access to such supports. (p. 35)

Competency 5: Facilitation of Services	The community support human service practitioner is knowledgeable about a range of participatory planning techniques and is skilled in implementing plans in a collaborative and expeditious manner. (p. 40)
Competency 6: Community and Living Skills and Supports	The community support human service practitioner has the ability to match specific supports and interventions to the unique needs of individual participants and recognizes the importance of friends, family and community relationships. (p. 45)
Competency 7: Education, Training, and Self-Development	The community support human service practitioner should be able to identify areas for self-improvement, pursue necessary educational/training resources, and share knowledge with others. (p. 51)
Competency 8: Advocacy	The community support human service practitioner should be knowledgeable about the diverse challenges facing participants (e.g., human rights, legal, administrative and financial) and should be able to identify and use effective advocacy strategies to overcome such challenges. (p. 54)
Competency 9: Vocational, Educational, and Career Support	The community support human service practitioner should be knowledgeable about the career and education related concerns of the participant and should be able to mobilize the resources and support necessary to assist the participant to reach his or her goals. (p. 57)
Competency 10: Crisis Intervention	The community support human service practitioner should be knowledgeable about crisis prevention, intervention and resolution techniques and should match such techniques to particular circumstances and individuals. (p. 60)
Competency 11: Organizational Participation	The community based support worker is familiar with the mission and practices of the support organization and participates in the life of the organization. (p. 63)
Competency 12: Documentation	The community based support worker is aware of the requirements for documentation in his or her organization and is able to manage these requirements efficiently. (p. 67)

SOURCE: Taylor, Bradly, & Warren, 1996.

Appendix B

Ethical Standards of Human Service Professionals

National Organization for Human Service Education

Council for Standards in Human Service Education

PREAMBLE

Human services is a profession developing in response to and in anticipation of the direction of human needs and human problems in the late twentieth century. Characterized particularly by an appreciation of human beings in all of their diversity, human services offers assistance to its clients within the context of their community and environment. Human service professionals, regardless of whether they are students, faculty or practitioners, promote and encourage the unique values and characteristics of human services. In so doing human service professionals uphold the integrity and ethics of the profession, partake in constructive criticism of the profession, promote client and community well-being, and enhance their own professional growth.

The ethical guidelines presented are a set of standards of conduct which the human service professional considers in ethical and professional decision making. It is hoped that these guidelines will be of assistance when the human service professional is challenged by difficult ethical dilemmas. Although ethical codes are not legal documents, they may be used to assist in the adjudication of issues related to ethical human service behavior.

SOURCE: From "Ethical Standards of Human Service Professionals," by National Organization of Human Service Education. Copyright © 1995 National Organization of Human Service Education. Reprinted with permission. Retrieved May 1, 2001, from the World Wide Web: http://nohse.com/ethstand.html

SECTION I—STANDARDS FOR HUMAN SERVICE PROFESSIONALS

Human service professionals function in many ways and carry out many roles. They enter into professional-client relationships with individuals, families, groups and communities who are all referred to as "clients" in these standards. Among their roles are caregiver, case manager, broker, teacher/educator, behavior changer, consultant, outreach professional, mobilizer, advocate, community planner, community change organizer, evaluator and administrator.[1.] The following standards are written with these multifaceted roles in mind.

THE HUMAN SERVICE PROFESSIONAL'S RESPONSIBILITY TO CLIENTS

Statement 1

Human service professionals negotiate with clients the purpose, goals, and nature of the helping relationship prior to its onset as well as inform clients of the limitations of the proposed relationship.

Statement 2

Human service professionals respect the integrity and welfare of the client at all times. Each client is treated with respect, acceptance and dignity.

Statement 3

Human service professionals protect the client's right to privacy and confidentiality except when such confidentiality would cause harm to the client or others, when agency guidelines state otherwise, or under other stated conditions (e.g., local, state, or federal laws). Professionals inform clients of the limits of confidentiality prior to the onset of the helping relationship.

Statement 4

If it is suspected that danger or harm may occur to the client or to others as a result of a client's behavior, the human service professional acts in an appropriate and professional manner to protect the safety of those individuals. This may involve seeking consultation, supervision, and/or breaking the confidentiality of the relationship.

Statement 5

Human service professionals protect the integrity, safety, and security of client records. All written client information that is shared with other professionals, except in the course of professional supervision, must have the client's prior written consent.

Statement 6

Human service professionals are aware that in their relationships with clients power and status are unequal. Therefore they recognize that dual or multiple relationships may increase the risk of harm to, or exploitation of, clients, and may impair their professional judgment. However, in some communities and situations it may not be feasible to avoid social or other nonprofessional contact with clients. Human service professionals support the trust implicit in the helping relationship by avoiding dual relationships that may impair professional judgment, increase the risk of harm to clients or lead to exploitation.

Statement 7

Sexual relationships with current clients are not considered to be in the best interest of the client and are prohibited. Sexual relationships with previous clients are considered dual relationships and are addressed in Statement 6 (above).

Statement 8

The client's right to self-determination is protected by human service professionals. They recognize the client's right to receive or refuse services.

Statement 9

Human service professionals recognize and build on client strengths.

THE HUMAN SERVICE PROFESSIONAL'S RESPONSIBILITY TO THE COMMUNITY AND SOCIETY

Statement 10

Human service professionals are aware of local, state, and federal laws. They advocate for change in regulations and statutes when such legislation conflicts with ethical guidelines and/or client rights. Where laws are harmful to individuals, groups or communities, human service professionals consider the conflict between the values of obeying the law and the values of serving people and may decide to initiate social action.

Statement 11

Human service professionals keep informed about current social issues as they affect the client and the community. They share that information with clients, groups and community as part of their work.

Statement 12

Human service professionals understand the complex interaction between individuals, their families, the communities in which they live, and society.

Statement 13

Human service professionals act as advocates in addressing unmet client and community needs. Human service professionals provide a mechanism for identifying unmet client needs, calling attention to these needs, and assisting in planning and mobilizing to advocate for those needs at the local community level.

Statement 14

Human service professionals represent their qualifications to the public accurately.

Statement 15

Human service professionals describe the effectiveness of programs, treatments, and/or techniques accurately.

Statement 16

Human service professionals advocate for the rights of all members of society, particularly those who are members of minorities and groups at which discriminatory practices have historically been directed.

Statement 17

Human service professionals provide services without discrimination or preference based on age, ethnicity, culture, race, disability, gender, religion, sexual orientation or socioeconomic status.

Statement 18

Human service professionals are knowledgeable about the cultures and communities within which they practice. They are aware of multiculturalism in society and its impact on the community as well as individuals within the community. They respect individuals and groups, their cultures and beliefs.

Statement 19

Human service professionals are aware of their own cultural backgrounds, beliefs, and values, recognizing the potential for impact on their relationships with others.

Statement 20

Human service professionals are aware of sociopolitical issues that differentially affect clients from diverse backgrounds.

Statement 21

Human service professionals seek the training, experience, education and supervision necessary to ensure their effectiveness in working with culturally diverse client populations.

THE HUMAN SERVICE PROFESSIONAL'S RESPONSIBILITY TO COLLEAGUES

Statement 22

Human service professionals avoid duplicating another professional's helping relationship with a client. They consult with other professionals who are assisting the client in a different type of relationship when it is in the best interest of the client to do so.

Statement 23

When a human service professional has a conflict with a colleague, he or she first seeks out the colleague in an attempt to manage the problem. If necessary, the professional then seeks the assistance of supervisors, consultants or other professionals in efforts to manage the problem.

Statement 24

Human service professionals respond appropriately to unethical behavior of colleagues. Usually this means initially talking directly with the colleague and, if no resolution is forthcoming, reporting the colleague's behavior to supervisory or administrative staff and/or to the professional organization(s) to which the colleague belongs.

Statement 25

All consultations between human service professionals are kept confidential unless to do so would result in harm to clients or communities.

THE HUMAN SERVICE PROFESSIONAL'S RESPONSIBILITY TO THE PROFESSION

Statement 26

Human service professionals know the limit and scope of their professional knowledge and offer services only within their knowledge and skill base.

Statement 27

Human service professionals seek appropriate consultation and supervision to assist in decision-making when there are legal, ethical or other dilemmas.

Statement 28

Human service professionals act with integrity, honesty, genuineness, and objectivity.

Statement 29

Human service professionals promote cooperation among related disciplines (e.g., psychology, counseling, social work, nursing, family and consumer sciences, medicine, education) to foster professional growth and interests within the various fields.

Statement 30

Human service professionals promote the continuing development of their profession. They encourage membership in professional associations, support research endeavors, foster educational advancement, advocate for appropriate legislative actions, and participate in other related professional activities.

Statement 31

Human service professionals continually seek out new and effective approaches to enhance their professional abilities.

THE HUMAN SERVICE PROFESSIONAL'S RESPONSIBILITY TO EMPLOYERS

Statement 32

Human service professionals adhere to commitments made to their employers.

Statement 33

Human service professionals participate in efforts to establish and maintain employment conditions which are conducive to high quality client services. They assist in evaluating the effectiveness of the agency through reliable and valid assessment measures.

Statement 34

When a conflict arises between fulfilling the responsibility to the employer and the responsibility to the client, human service professionals advise both of the conflict and work conjointly with all involved to manage the conflict.

THE HUMAN SERVICE PROFESSIONAL'S RESPONSIBILITY TO SELF

Statement 35

Human service professionals strive to personify those characteristics typically associated with the profession (e.g., accountability, respect for others, genuineness, empathy, pragmatism).

Statement 36

Human service professionals foster self-awareness and personal growth in themselves. They recognize that when professionals are aware of their own values, attitudes, cultural background, and personal needs, the process of helping others is less likely to be negatively impacted by those factors.

Statement 37

Human service professionals recognize a commitment to lifelong learning and continually upgrade knowledge and skills to serve the populations better.

SECTION II—STANDARDS FOR HUMAN SERVICE EDUCATORS

Human Service educators are familiar with, informed by, and accountable to the standards of professional conduct put forth by their institutions of higher learning; their professional disciplines, for example, American Association of University Professors (AAUP), American Counseling Association (ACA), Academy of Criminal Justice (ACJS), American Psychological Association (APA), American Sociological Association (ASA), National Association of Social Workers (NASW), National Board of Certified Counselors (NBCC), National Education Association (NEA); and the National Organization for Human Service Education (NOHSE).

Statement 38

Human service educators uphold the principle of liberal education and embrace the essence of academic freedom, abstaining from inflicting their own personal views/morals on students, and allowing students the freedom to express their views without penalty, censure, or ridicule, and to engage in critical thinking.

Statement 39

Human service educators provide students with readily available and explicit program policies and criteria regarding program goals and objectives, recruitment, admission, course requirements, evaluations, retention, and dismissal in accordance with due process procedures.

Statement 40

Human service educators demonstrate high standards of scholarship in content areas and of pedagogy by staying current with developments in the field of Human Services and in teaching effectiveness, such as learning styles and teaching styles.

Statement 41

Human service educators monitor students' field experiences to ensure the quality of the placement site, supervisory experience, and learning experience towards the goals of professional identity and skill development.

Statement 42

Human service educators participate actively in the selection of required reading and use them with care, based strictly on the merits of the material's content, and present relevant information accurately, objectively and fully.

Statement 43

Human service educators, at the onset of courses: inform students if sensitive/controversial issues or experiential/affective content or process are part of the course design; ensure that students are offered opportunities to discuss in structured ways their reactions to sensitive or controversial class content; ensure that the presentation of such material is justified on pedagogical grounds directly related to the course; and, differentiate between information based on scientific data, anecdotal data, and personal opinion.

Statement 44

Human service educators develop and demonstrate culturally sensitive knowledge, awareness, and teaching methodology.

Statement 45

Human service educators demonstrate full commitment to their appointed responsibilities and are enthusiastic about and encouraging of students' learning.

Statement 46

Human service educators model the personal attributes, values, and skills of the human service professional, including, but not limited to, the willingness to seek and respond to feedback from students.

Statement 47

Human service educators establish and uphold appropriate guidelines concerning self-disclosure or student-disclosure of sensitive/personal information.

Statement 48

Human service educators establish an appropriate and timely process for providing clear and objective feedback to students about their performance on relevant and established course/program academic and personal competence requirements and their suitability for the field.

Statement 49

Human service educators are aware that in their relationships with students, power and status are unequal; therefore, human service educators are responsible to clearly define and maintain ethical and professional relationships with students, and avoid conduct that is demeaning, embarrassing or exploitative of students, and to treat students fairly, equally and without discrimination.

Statement 50

Human service educators recognize and acknowledge the contributions of students to their work, for example in case material, workshops, research, publications.

Statement 51

Human service educators demonstrate professional standards of conduct in managing personal or professional differences with colleagues, for example, not disclosing such differences and/or affirming a student's negative opinion of a faculty/program.

Statement 52

Human service educators ensure that students are familiar with, informed by, and accountable to the ethical standards and policies put forth by their program/department, the course syllabus/instructor, their advisor(s), and the Ethical Standards of Human Service Professionals.

Statement 53

Human service educators are aware of all relevant curriculum standards, including those of the Council for Standards in Human Services Education (CSHSE); the Community Support Skills Standards; and state/local standards, and take them into consideration in designing the curriculum.

Statement 54

Human service educators create a learning context in which students can achieve the knowledge, skills, values and attitudes of the academic program.

[1.] Southern Regional Education Board. (1967). Roles and Functions of Mental Health Workers: A Report of a Symposium. Atlanta, GA: Community Mental Health Worker Project.

Appendix C

Summary of Goals, Skills, and Attitudes of the Stages of the Helping Relationship and Exercises Associated with Them

Below is a summary of some of the skills that might be used at the various stages of helping. After reviewing the skills, complete the exercise associated with each stage.

Summary of Goals, Skills, and Attitudes of the Stages of the Helping Relationship*

Stage	Goals	Skills/Attitudes
Pre-Interview	a. Complete paperwork b. Set tone c. Complete intake interview	a. Courteousness b. Being cordial c. Gathering information

Stage 1:
Rapport and
Trust Building
	a. Develop safe atmosphere
	b. Give professional
	   disclosure statement
	c. Obtain informed consent
	d. Make preliminary assessment
	   and diagnosis
		a. Cordiality
		b. Good social skills
		c. Listening skills
		d. Empathy skills

Stage 2:
Problem
Identification
	a. Validate initial assessment
	   and diagnosis
	b. Change assessment and
	   diagnosis as necessary
		a. Higher level empathy
		b. Questions
		c. Affirmation
		d. Encouragement
		e. Self-disclosure

Stage 3: Goal Setting	a. Collaboratively set general and/or specific goals	a. Listening b. Empathy c. Information giving d. Feedback e. Offering advice f. Offering alternatives g. Affirming

(Continued)

Continued

Stage	Goals	Skills/Attitudes
Stage 4: Work	a. Work on identified goals b. Clarify goals, if necessary c. Set new goals, if necessary	a. Confrontation b. Probing questions c. Self-disclosure d. Advanced empathy e. Modeling f. Affirmation g. Encouragement h. Specialized skills
Stage 5: Closure	a. Summarize progress b. Review met goals c. Discuss feelings about ending d. Tie up loose ends	a. Summarizing b. Listening c. Empathy d. Self-disclosure
Stage 6: Post-Interview: The Revolving Door	a. Assure client satisfaction b. Assure change has been maintained c. Assess effectiveness of helping relationship d. Reinforce past change e. Set up additional appointments or referrals	a. Cordial telephone contact b. Effective letter writing c. Effective survey development d. Knowledge of referrals

*Note: The characteristics of the effective helper should be embodied throughout the stages.

The following group of exercises can be completed one at a time, or they can be treated as one seamless exercise. This group of exercises is likely to take a whole class period.

EXERCISE 1 The Pre-Interview Stage

This exercise can be done with the whole class or in small groups. The instructor, or students who have worked at an agency, may want to bring some samples of paperwork that clients complete when first entering an agency. The instructor may want to rearrange the classroom so it has more of an agency waiting room feel. Next, the instructor should identify a fictitious "agency" a client will enter. Then, a student will volunteer to role-play a client who will be assigned to a role-play helper. A role-play secretary should also be identified. The secretary should discuss with the instructor the process the client will go through at the agency. The secretary will later explain this process to the client.

The client will walk into the agency and make initial contact with the secretary. The secretary will then explain to the client the process he or she will go through at the agency and give any paperwork to the client. When the paperwork is completed, the secretary will refer the client to a helper to complete any additional paperwork and complete a structured interview as delineated in Chapter 6. After the gathering of information is completed, the client can be referred to a second helper for counseling or remain with the same helper. When the exercise is complete, answer the following questions:

1. Did the client feel comfortable in this agency?
2. Could the client have been treated in a more humane fashion?
3. Was the process effective for gathering preliminary data from the client?
4. Did the client have a feel for what was going to happen to him or her?
5. Are there any other suggestions for making this process better?

EXERCISE 2   Stage 1: Rapport and Trust-Building

In small groups identify two students, one to role-play a client and one to role-play a helper. Have the helper and client role-play the first stage of the helping relationship. Make sure the client is given a professional disclosure statement and gives informed consent. Also make sure the helper uses his or her basic listening skills to build a relationship and obtain an initial assessment of the problem. After role-playing for approximately 15 minutes, the small group should offer feedback to the helper. The following questions might assist in that process:

1. Was the helper cordial and friendly?
2. Did the helper give the client a professional disclosure statement?
3. Did the helper obtain informed consent?
4. Did the helper mostly use his or her foundational skills in building a relationship?
5. Did the helper avoid the use of other skills (e.g., helper-centered skills) at this point of the relationship?
6. Did the helper summarize what he or she had learned from the client at the end of the stage and make a preliminary assessment and/or diagnosis?

EXERCISE 3   Stage 2: Problem-Identification

Proceed with the same situation as earlier, but have two new students continue with the role-play. Using the information above, the helper and client should continue to probe to assure that the assessment of the problem is accurate. Do this for approximately 10 minutes and then answer the following questions:

1. Was the helper able to maintain a trusting relationship even though he or she was now asking questions and probing further?
2. Did the initial assessment of the client problem change?
3. Is the helper prepared to begin the goal-setting process, or is more probing and clarification necessary?

EXERCISE 4   Stage 3: The Goal-Setting

Continuing with the same situation, but changing the helper and client, role-play the goal-setting stage. Do this for approximately 10 minutes and then respond to the questions below:

1. What techniques did the helper use to assist the client in setting goals?
2. Were the techniques used helpful in setting goals or would other techniques have been better?
3. Were the goals chosen in a collaborative fashion?
4. Are the chosen goals reasonable considering the information that was obtained in the previous stages?
5. Are the chosen goals attainable?

EXERCISE 5   Stage 4: Work

Continuing with the same situation as earlier, but changing the helper and client, role-play the work stage with the client. Do this for approximately 10 minutes and then respond to the questions below:

1. Was the helper able to identify whether the client had worked successfully on his or her identified goals?
2. What skills did the helper employ, and in what manner, to assure that the client is working toward his or her goals?
3. Were there other techniques that might have been helpful for the helper to use?

EXERCISE 6   Stage 5: Closure

Continuing with the same situation, but changing the helper and client, role-play the closure stage with the client. Do this for approximately 10 minutes and then respond to the questions below:

1. Did the helper summarize the progress the client has made and affirm his or her positive steps toward change?
2. Did the helper give the client an opportunity to discuss how he or she feels about ending the helping relationship?
3. Did the helper share feelings about the ending of the helping relationship?
4. Did the helper make sure that there was a sense of an "ending" and that new issues did not arise?

Appendix D

Overview of *DSM-IV-TR* Diagnoses

TYPES OF DISORDERS (BASED ON *DSM-IV-TR*)

DSM-IV-TR offers a wealth of information on disorders that is used by clinicians in making sound diagnostic judgments. The following summarizes hundreds of pages of information from Axis I and Axis II of DSM-IV-TR.

BRIEF OVERVIEW OF AXIS I DISORDERS

Disorders Usually First Diagnosed in Infancy, Childhood, or Adolescence: The disorders in this section are generally found in childhood, however, at times individuals are not diagnosed with the disorder until they are adults. The diagnosis, however, can still be made and classified on Axis I. This does not include, however, mental retardation, which is diagnosed on Axis II. The following disorders, which are particularly important for helpers who work with children, are found in this section:

Learning Disorders: Used when a child's academic functioning is substantially below the child's age, intelligence, and education level. They include Reading Disorder, Mathematics Disorder, Disorder of Written Expression, and Learning Disorder Not Otherwise Specified.

Motor Skills Disorder: Includes Developmental Coordination Disorder, when motor coordination is substantially below what is expected.

Communication Disorders: Characterized by difficulties in speech or language. Includes Expressive Language Disorder, Mixed Receptive-Expressive Language Disorder, Phonological Disorder, Stuttering, and Communication Disorder Not Otherwise Specified.

Pervasive Developmental Disorders: These disorders are characterized by pervasive developmental deficits in many areas. They include Autistic Disorder, Rett's Disorder, Childhood Disintegrative Disorder, Asperger's Disorder, and Pervasive Developmental Disorder Not Otherwise Specified.

Attention-Deficit and Disruptive Behavior Disorders: This section includes the Attention Deficit Disorders characterized by inattention and/or hyperactivity-impulsivity; Conduct Disorder, characterized by inappropriate behavior and violation of the basic rights of others; and Oppositional Defiant Disorder, characterized by negative, hostile, and defiant behavior.

Feeding and Eating Disorders of Infancy or Early Childhood: Characterized by ongoing disturbances in feeding and eating, these disorders include Pica (eating nonnutritious substances such as plaster, hair, insects, animal droppings), Rumination Disorder (regurgitation and rechewing of food), and Feeding Disorder of Infancy or Early Childhood (failure to eat with no apparent medical condition).

Tic Disorders: Characterized by vocal and/or motor tics, these disorders include Tourette's Disorder, Chronic Motor or Vocal Tic Disorder, Transient Tic Disorder, and Tic Disorder Not Otherwise Specified.

Elimination Disorders: Encopresis (repeated passage of feces into inappropriate places) and Enuresis (repeated voiding of urine into inappropriate places) are the two disorders associated with Elimination Disorders.

Other Disorders of Infancy, Childhood, or Adolescence: This section is for disorders not included in the other groupings. They include Separation Anxiety, Selective Mutism (failure to speak in selective situations), Reactive Attachment Disorder of Infancy or Early Childhood (disturbed social relatedness due to pathological caretaking), Stereotypic Movement Disorder (e.g., headbanging, arm flailing, and so forth, which could result in bodily harm), and Disorders of Infancy, Childhood, or Adolescence Not Otherwise Specified.

Delirium, Dementia, Amnestic, and Other Cognitive Disorders: Delirium, dementia and anmestic disorders are all cognitive disorders that represent a significant change from past cognitive functioning of the client. All of these disorders are caused by a medical condition or a substance (e.g., drug abuse, medication, allergic reaction).

Delirium is characterized by a confused mental state that may include disorientation, delusions, hallucinations, unconsciousness, and sometimes memory loss. Dementia often involves the atrophy of brain tissue and the resulting development of multiple cognitive deficits that can include memory impairment, aphasia, deterioration of language functioning, apraxia, impaired ability to execute motor activities, poor judgment, and disorientation. Individuals with an Amnestic Disorder have memory impairment without delirium or confusion, are unable to learn new material or remember past information.

Mental Disorders Due to a General Medical Condition: This diagnosis is made when a mental disorder is found to be directly related to a medical condition, such as a person who hallucinates as the result of a brain tumor. Three classes of disorders due to a medical condition are noted in this section and include catatonic disorder, personality change, and mental disorder not otherwise specified. Other disorders due to a medical condition can be found in specific diagnostic categories (e.g., psychotic disorder due to a general medical condition would be found under "psychotic disorders").

Substance-Related Disorders: A substance-related disorder is a direct result of the use of a drug or alcohol, the effects of medication, or exposure to a toxin. Substances are classified into 11 groups that include alcohol; amphetamines; caffeine; cannabis; cocaine; hallucinogens; inhalants; nicotine; opioids; phencyclidine (PCP); and sedatives, hypnotics, or anxiolytics. Also included are polysubstance dependence and Other or Unknown Substance-Related Disorders. The DSM-IV-TR differentiates between Substance Dependence, Substance Abuse, and Substance-Induced Disorders.

Schizophrenia and Other Psychotic Disorders: All disorders classified in this section have in common psychotic symptomology as their most distinguishing feature. A broad definition of psychosis would include some or all of the following symptoms: delusions, hallucinations, incoherence, disorganized thinking, disorganized speech, disorganized or catatonic behavior, and a loss of contact with reality. A number of disorders that share different aspects of the above can be found in this section and include schizophrenia, shizophreniform disorder, schizoaffective disorder, delusional disorder, brief psychotic disorder, shared psychotic disorder, psychotic disorder due to a general medication condition, substance-induced psychotic disorder, and psychotic disorder not otherwise specified.

Mood Disorders: The disorders in this category share a common feature—mood disturbances of the depressive, manic, or hypomanic type. Mood disorders of the depressive type are characterized by extreme depressive features, feelings of low self-esteem, poor appetite and overeating, poor concentration, low energy and fatigue, suicidal thoughts, significant weight loss, and serious problems in social and occupational functioning. Those exhibiting hypomanic episodes show such symptoms as inflated self-esteem and grandiosity, decreased need for sleep, distractibility and flight of ideas, involvement in pleasurable activities that may cause serious negative consequences, but no psychotic features or serious problems in social or occupational functioning. In manic episodes, besides the above symptoms, psychosis and serious disturbances at work or with social functioning may occur.

The Mood Disorders are divided into three broad categories: (1) the Depressive Disorders, which are characterized by a depressed mood and no manic or hypomanic episodes (e.g., Major-Depressive Disorder, Dysthymic Disorder, and Depressive Disorder not Otherwise Specified), (2) the Bipolar Disorders, which are characterized by depression and manic or hypomanic episodes (e.g., Bipolar I and II Disorders, Cyclothymic Disorder, and Bipolar Disorder Not

Otherwise Classified), and (3) the Other Mood Disorders, which are Mood Disorders Related to a General Medication Condition, a Substance-Induced Mood Disorder, or a Mood Disorder Not Otherwise Specified.

Anxiety Disorders: There are many types of Anxiety Disorders, each with its own discrete characteristics. They include (1) Panic Attack: the sudden onset of fear and severe terror not related to any obviously threatening situation, (2) Agoraphobia: fear of places or situations, (3) Panic Disorder With or Without Agoraphobia: persistent unexpected panic attacks either with, or without agoraphobia, (4) Agoraphobia Without History of Panic Disorder: symptoms of agoraphobia but no panic-like symptoms as would be found in a panic disorder, (5) Specific Phobia: extreme anxiety related to a specific situation, (6) Obsessive-Compulsive Disorder: obsessions that cause extreme anxiety and compulsions (e.g., hand washing) to neutralize the anxiety, (7) Posttraumatic Stress Disorder: reexperiencing of a traumatic event leading to extreme anxiety, (8) Acute Stress Disorder: extreme anxiety appearing directly following an acutely traumatic event, (9) Generalized Anxiety Disorder: persistent anxiety lasting a minimum of six months, (10) Anxiety Disorder Due to a General Medical Condition: anxiety as a direct response to a medical condition, (11) Substance-Induced Anxiety Disorder: anxiety as a direct response to drug abuse, medication, or toxin; (12) Anxiety Disorder Not Otherwise Specified: other anxiety symptoms that do not fall into any of the previous categories.

Somatoform Disorders: Somatoform disorders are characterized by symptoms that would suggest a physical cause; however, no such cause can be found, and there is strong evidence that links the symptoms to psychological causes. In somatoform disorders the symptoms cause significant psychological distress or serious impairment to social and/or occupational functioning. Seven somatoform disorders listed in DSM-IV-TR include (1) Somatization Disorder: physical symptoms that begin before age 30 and extend for years and include pain, gastrointestinal, sexual, and pseudoneurological symptoms, (2) Undifferentiated Somatoform Disorder: a physical complaint that occurs for six months or longer for which no medical reason can be found, (3) Conversion Disorder: symptoms presented by the client seem to suggest a neurological condition, but upon laboratory testing, there is no explainable cause, (4) Pain Disorder: pain at one or more anatomical sites that appears to be related to psychological factors, (5) Hypochondriasis: a preoccupation that one has a serious illness when none indeed exist, (6) Body Dysmorphic Disorder: a preoccupation with an imagined defect in the person's appearance when indeed no major defect is present, and (7) Somatoform Disorder Not Otherwise Specified: other disorders of a somatoform nature not covered under the previous diagnoses.

Factitious Disorders: As opposed to Somatoform Disorders, which describe individuals who believe that their physical symptoms have a physiological etiology, Factitious Disorders describe individuals who intentionally feign physical or psychological symptoms in order to assume the "sick role." As opposed to malingering, which occurs when the individual consciously fakes a symptom for an external secondary gain ("I don't want to go to work so I'll call in sick"), Factitious Disorders fulfill a psychological need and are not used for an obvious external gain. In these disorders, physical symptoms may or may not actually be present. Two subtypes of this disorder are Factitious Disorder with Predominantly Psychological Signs and Symptoms, and Factitious Disorder With Predominantly Physical Signs and Symptoms. One interesting manifestation of this latter type is Munchausen's Syndrome, in which the individual spends most of his or her life feigning illnesses with the purpose of getting admitted to a hospital. Munchausen's Syndrome by Proxy describes a parent who intentionally poisons or harms his or her child in an effort to have his or her child immediately hospitalized.

Dissociative Disorders: Dissociative Disorders involve a disruption of consciousness, memory, identity, or perception of the environment. Five dissociative disorders are (1) Dissociative Amnesia: inability to remember important personal information that cannot be attributed to normal forgetfulness, (2) Dissociative Fugue: an unconscious flight from reality when the individual leaves his or her current environment and takes on a new, fully functioning normal life, while having no ability to recall the past life, (3) Dissociative Identity Disorder, formerly called Multiple Personality Disorder: taking on two or more unique personalities that generally have little knowledge of one another, (4) Depersonalization Disorder: persistent feelings of being out of touch with reality or a sense of detachment from self, and (5) Dissociative Disorder Not Otherwise Specified: disorders whose prominent features are of a dissociative nature but cannot be classified in one of the previous categories.

Sexual and Gender Identity Disorders: This section includes Sexual Dysfunctions, Paraphilias, Gender Identity Disorders, and Sexual Disorder Not Otherwise Specified. Sexual Dysfunctions include those disorders in which there is a disturbance of sexual desire that causes the individual severe distress and problems in relationships. The disorders may be psychologically caused or caused by a combination of psychological and physical factors (e.g., pain upon erection due to a disease may lead to lack of sexual desire even though the individual can ejaculate).

The Sexual Dysfunction Disorders include Sexual Desire Disorders, Sexual Arousal Disorders, Orgasmic Disorders, Sexual Pain Disorders, Sexual Dysfunction Due to a General Medical Condition, Substance-Induced Sexual Dysfunction, and Sexual Dysfunction Not Otherwise Specified.

Paraphilia includes those disorders that are characterized by sexual urges, fantasies, or behaviors toward inappropriate partners, unusual objects, activities, or situations along with clinically significant distress or impairment in social, occupational, or other important areas of functioning. They include Exhibitionism, Fetishism, Frotteurism, Pedophilia, Masochism, Sadism, Transvestism, Voyeurism, and Paraphilia Not Otherwise Specified.

Gender Identity Disorders include those disorders in which an individual will have a strong identification with and desire to be the gender different from his or her biological sex.

Eating Disorders: There are three diagnoses within this category, all of which are considered severe forms of eating disorders. They include Anorexia Nervosa, Bulimia Nervosa, and Eating Disorder Not Otherwise Specified.

In Anorexia Nervosa the individual is extremely fearful of gaining weight and has a perceptual disturbance of body size and/or shape. In Anorexia there is extreme weight loss usually resulting from self-starvation, excessive exercise, and/or over-compensatory self-regulatory behaviors such as binge eating and purging, and laxative, diuretic, or enema misuse. Anorexics can be either restrictive eaters or binge-eating/purge types.

Like Anorexics, Bulimics are overly concerned with body shape and size and may have a distorted image of their body. Bulimics tend to binge eat regularly, eating quantities much larger than the usual person would eat. This is followed by methods to prevent weight gain such as misuse of laxatives, diuretics, enemas, vomiting, fasting, and exercise. Bulimics can be of the purge or non-purge types. To qualify for this diagnosis, the binge eating and other behaviors must occur at least three times per week for at least three months.

The last category, Eating Disorder Not Otherwise Specified, includes other eating disorders not included in Anorexia or Bulimia.

Sleep Disorders: The Sleep Disorders are broken down into four subcategories: Primary Sleep Disorders, Sleep Disorder Related to Another Mental Condition, Sleep Disorder Due to a General Medical Condition, and Substance-Induced Sleep Disorder.

Primary Sleep Disorders are of two types: Dyssomnias and Parasomnias. Dyssomnias are characterized by difficulty going to sleep, staying asleep, or being excessively tired. Dyssomnias include Primary Insomnia, Primary Hypersomnia (sleeping too much and still being tired), Narcolepsy (irresistible sleep attacks), Breathing-Related Sleep Disorder (sleep disruption due to a breathing condition), Circadian Rhythm Sleep Disorder (sleep-related problems due to an unavoidable inability to sleep during the individual's natural sleep patterns), and Dyssomnia Not Otherwise Specified.

Parasomnias are different from the Dyssomnias in that individuals suffering from these disorders do not have any abnormalities in the sleep-wake cycle. Instead, the autonomic nervous system is activated at unpredictable times. Probably the most common disorder is Nightmare Disorder, but others include Sleep Terror Disorder (recurrent, abrupt, fearful awakening not associated with a dream), Sleepwalking Disorder, and Parasomnia Not Otherwise Specified.

Impulse Control Disorders Not Elsewhere Classified: Since many other mental disorders are associated with a lack of impulse control, this section examines only those impulse control disorders not classified under other mental disorders. Impulse Control Disorders are underscored by an intense uncontrollable arousal to commit an impulsive act followed by feelings of pleasure, gratification, and relief while committing the act. There may or may not be guilt or regret following the act. The primary disorders in this section are Intermittent Explosive Disorder, Kleptomania, Pyromania, Pathological Gambling, Trichotillomania (pulling out one's hair), and Impulse-Control Disorder Not Otherwise Specified.

Adjustment Disorders: Adjustment disorders are probably the most common disorders clinicians see in private practice. Adjustment disorders are distinguished by emotional or behavioral symptoms that arise in response to psychosocial stressors. To be classified as an adjustment disorder such symptoms must have developed within three months of exposure to the stressor and should dissipate within six months unless the stressor is chronic (e.g., chronic prostatitis).

A number of subtypes of Adjustment Disorders exist including Adjustment Disorders with depressed mood, with anxiety, with mixed anxiety and depressed mood, with disturbance of conduct, with mixed disturbance of emotions and conduct, and unspecified.

BRIEF OVERVIEW OF AXIS II DISORDERS

Mental Retardation: Characterized by intellectual functioning significantly below average (at least two standard deviations below the mean on intelligence tests—below the 2nd percentile), mental retardation can have many different etiologies. There are four categories of mental retardation: Mild Mental Retardation (IQ of 50–55 to approximately 70), Moderate Mental Retardation (IQ of 35–40 to 50–55), Severe Mental Retardation (IQ of 20–25 to 35–40), and Profound Mental Retardation (IQ level below 20 or 25).

Personality Disorders: Personality Disorders are characterized by patterns of relating to the world that are deeply ingrained, inflexible and enduring; they deviate from what is considered usual ways of relating. Individuals with this type of disorder may have difficulty understanding self and others, may be labile, may have difficulty in relationships, and may have problems with impulse control. Personality disorders are generally first recognized in adolescence or early adulthood and often remain throughout one's lifetime. They lead to distress and impairment in the person's life. As noted earlier, there are three clusters of personality disorders, and one other category "Personality Disorder Not Otherwise Specified" for personality disorders that do not fit into any of the three clusters.

Cluster A includes Paranoid, Schizoid, and Schizotypal Personality Disorder. Individuals with these disorders all experience and display characteristics that may be considered odd or eccentric by others. Individuals with Paranoid Personality Disorder are suspicious, hypersensitive, and mistrustful people. Individuals with Schizoid Personality Disorder are generally loners; they are shy, are restrictive in emotion, lack warmth and empathy, and are indifferent to how others feel about them. Individuals with Schizotypal Personality Disorder lack social and interpersonal skills, have little ability to form relationships, are eccentric, and have distorted views of the world. They tend to have odd thoughts, may talk to themselves, and be difficult to follow; their affect is flat.

Cluster B disorders include the Antisocial, Borderline, Histrionic, and Narcissistic Personality Disorders. Individuals suffering from these disorders are generally dramatic, emotional, overly sensitive, and erratic. "Why do I rob banks? Because that is where the money is," describes an individual suffering from Antisocial Personality Disorder. Antisocial individuals have little regard for the rights of others, do not conform to social norms, may not respect laws, are irresponsible, and will impulsively harm others and have little or no remorse. Borderline personalities may impulsively use drugs, have sex, and spend money; they may binge eat and/or drive recklessly. Such individuals will likely have difficulty maintaining a stable relationship and may be suicidal or self-mutilating, have emotional swings, and feel chronically empty inside. Histrionic individuals are lively, are overly dramatic, and always call attention to themselves. They have frequent emotional outbursts, are quickly bored, and desire stimulation and excitement. The individual with a Narcissistic Personality Disorder always wants attention. "You're so vain, you probably think this song is about you" describes the narcissistic person. He or she is preoccupied with self, intolerant of criticism, and grandiose; has a sense of entitlement; and believes that he or she is special in the world and capable of unlimited success, power, and status.

Cluster C includes the Avoidant, Dependent, and Obsessive Compulsive Personality Disorders. Common characteristics found within this cluster are anxious and fearful traits. Individuals with an Avoidant Personality Disorder are reticent to become involved in intimate relationships, socially withdrawn, fearful of rejection, and reluctant to take risks; they view themselves as socially inept and unappealing. Individuals who have a Dependent Personality Disorder are passive, are fearful of taking responsibility for their lives, lack self-confidence, cannot function independently, are submissive and clinging, and have a fear of separation. Orderliness, perfectionism, extreme control over their lives, overly involved with details, inflexible, and efficient are some of the words that describe the individual with an Obsessive-Compulsive Personality Disorder. These individuals are highly productive but rarely enjoy what they produce due to their perfectionistic stance in life.

OTHER CONDITIONS THAT MAY BE A FOCUS
OF CLINICAL ATTENTION

This section of DSM-IV-TR covers conditions or problems not listed on Axis I or Axis II and that fall into one of three general categories: (1) the presenting problem is the focus of the helping relationship but is not serious enough to require a diagnosis of a mental disorder, (2) the individual has a mental disorder but it is not the focus of treatment (e.g., an individual is Bipolar and seeks treatment for relational problems unrelated to the Bipolar disorder), and (3) an individual has a mental disorder that is related to a specific problem (an individual is Bipolar and the mental illness is causing relational problems that justify an adjustment disorder diagnosis). The specific problem is not considered a mental disorder but is serious enough to be the focus of clinical attention. A few examples of the many conditions that are included within this DSM-IV-TR section are Psychological Factors Affecting Medical Condition, Medication-Induced Movement Disorders, Other Medication Induced Disorders, Relational Problems, Problems Related to Abuse or Neglect, and Additional Conditions That May Be a Focus of Clinical Attention. For examples of any of the above listed disorders, the DSM-IV-TR should be consulted.

Appendix E

Global Assessment
of Functioning (GAF) Scale

Code	(Note: Use intermediate codes when appropriate, e.g., 45, 68, 72)
100 | 91	**Superior functioning in a wide range of activities, life's problems never seem to get out of hand, is sought out by others because of his or her many positive qualities. No symptoms.**
90 | 81	**Absent or minimal symptoms** (e.g., mild anxiety before an exam), **good functioning in all areas, interested and involved in a wide range of activities, socially effective, generally satisfied with life, no more than everyday problems or concerns** (e.g., an occasional argument with family members).
80 | 71	**If symptoms are present, they are transient and expectable reactions to psychosocial stressors** (e.g., difficulty concentrating after family argument); **no more than slight impairment in social, occupational, or school functioning** (e.g., temporarily falling behind in schoolwork).
70 | 61	**Some mild symptoms** (e.g., depressed mood and mild insomnia). **OR some difficulty in social, occupational or school functioning** (e.g., occasional truancy, or theft within the household), **but generally functioning pretty well, has some meaningful interpersonal relationships.**
60 | 51	**Moderate symptoms** (e.g., flat affect and circumstantial speech, occasional panic attacks). **OR some difficulty in social, occupational, or school functioning** (e.g., few friends, conflicts with peers or or co-workers).
50 | 41	**Serious symptoms** (e.g., suicidal ideation, severe obsessional rituals, frequent shoplifting) **OR any serious impairment in social occupational, or school functioning** (e.g., no friends, unable to keep a job).
40 | 31	**Some impairment in reality testing or communication** (e.g., speech is at times illogical, obscure, or or irrelevant) **OR major impairment in several areas, such as work or school, family relations, judgment, thinking, or mood** (e.g., depressed man avoids friends, neglects family, and is unable to work; child frequently beats up younger children, is defiant at home, and is failing at school).
30 | 21	**Behavior is considerably influenced by delusions or hallucinations OR serious impairment in communication or judgment** (e.g., sometimes incoherent, acts grossly inappropriately, suicidal preoccupation) **OR inability to function in almost all areas** (e.g., stays in bed all day; no job, home, or friends).
20 | 11	**Some danger of hurting self or others** (e.g., suicide attempts without clear expectation of death; frequently violent; manic excitement) **OR occasionally fails to maintain minimal personal hygiene** (e.g., smears feces) **OR gross impairment in communication** (e.g., largely incoherent or mute).
10 | 1	**Persistent danger of severely hurting self or others** (e.g., recurrent violence) **OR persistent inability to maintain minimal personal hygiene OR serious suicidal act with clear expectation of death.**
0	Inadequate information

SOURCE: *Diagnostic and Statistical Manual of Mental Disorders,* text revision (Fourth Edition). Copyright © 2000 American Psychiatric Association. Reprinted with permission.

Appendix F

Four Case Studies

Gloria

Gloria is a 53-year-old individual with a developmental disability. Gloria was born mildly mentally retarded and with cerebral palsy, and soon after her birth, her parents hospitalized her in an institution for the developmentally disabled. She lived in this institution until she was 31, at which time she was placed in a group home for the mentally retarded.

As a child, Gloria's language development was delayed. She could not speak in sentences until she was 4 years old. She was not toilet trained until age 7. Although her parents would visit her periodically, her main caretakers were the social service workers at the institution. Gloria was schooled at the institution where she acquired the equivalent of a second-grade education. Gloria had few friends in the institution and was considered a loner. Despite working on socialization skills while in the institution, Gloria still prefers to be alone and spends much of her time painting. She has become a rather good artist, and many of her paintings are found in the institution and in the group home. Visitors often comment on the paintings and are generally surprised that a developmentally disabled person can paint so well. Gloria has a part-time job at a local art-supply company where she generally does menial work.

Although Gloria does have some friends at the group home and at the art-supply store, generally, when she spends much time with someone, she ends up having a temper tantrum. When this happens, she will usually withdraw—often to her painting. Gloria generally blames other people for her anger.

Gloria is a rules follower. She feels very strongly about the list of rules on the bulletin board at her group home. She methodically reports people who break the rules. She always feels extremely guilty after having a temper tantrum because she sees herself as breaking the rule "talk things out rather than get into a fight." In a similar vein, Gloria feels that laws in the country "are there for a purpose." For instance, at street crossings she always stops at red lights and waits for the light to change.

Gloria has no sense of her future. She lives from day to day, and despite periods of depression, generally functions fairly adequately. She states she wants to get married, but her lack of socialization skills prevents her from having any meaningful relationships with men.

Overall, the human service workers who have contact with Gloria describe her as a rigid, conscientious, talented person who has trouble maintaining relationships. They note that despite being in individual counseling and in a socialization support group, she has made little progress in maintaining satisfying relationships. Their feeling is that she probably will maintain her current level of functioning, and they see little hope for change.

David

David is 13 years old and the only child, grandchild, or niece/nephew on his mother's side of the family. David's parents separated when his mother was five months pregnant with him. His parents, both of whom are highly educated, went through a tumultuous separation and divorce but now have a cordial relationship. Following his birth, his mother was distraught over the breakup of her marriage but subsequently has maintained a strong sense of self and high self-esteem. Following David's birth, his mother, who works full-time, was fortunately able to afford a live-in nanny. This woman still lives with them and has been a significant help for the family and an additional source of comfort for David.

David's mother remarried when David was 10 years old and his father has been involved in a long-term relationship. David lives with his mother but spends every other weekend, some weekdays, and extended periods of time during the summer and holidays with his father. He seems to have a good relationship with both parents, his stepfather, and his father's girlfriend.

David, who has always done well in school, currently attends a private school. He maintains very high grades and has a high IQ. David is at ease in relationships, as evidenced by his many friends and his ability to relate to people of all ages. He has many skills and is just beginning to examine those things that he is best at. He is just entering puberty, and girls are becoming more important to him. Overall, most people would describe David as a bright, personable, and thoughtful young man who is at ease with himself.

Although sometimes he may appear a little "spoiled," he generally is thoughtful and can recognize other people's feelings. He can think abstractly, and it would not be difficult to have a conversation with him concerning such philosophical matters as death and the existence of God.

Jason

Jason Reunter, 13, was brought in for counseling by his father because of Jason's feelings of depression and a drop in his grades within the last six months. He is the oldest of three children, having two younger sisters: Nicole who is 10 and Stephanie who is 7. Jason has been diagnosed as having Attention Deficit Disorder with Hyperactivity and Dyslexia. Until recently Jason obtained mostly As and Bs in school. Now, he is obtaining mostly Cs in school. Jason has over the years received assistance in a resource room for a math learning disability. Jason tends to be very well spoken and alert; he is described by teachers as "intellectually sharp." Jason has a fear of doctors and counselors, which his father relates to Jason's being treated for meningitis when he was four years old. The meningitis was successfully treated.

Jason's father, who is divorced, notes that he had always been satisfied in his marriage and was surprised when a couple of years ago his wife noted that she was unhappy. One year ago he and his wife separated and they recently were divorced. Mr. Reunter believes his wife left him in order to "discover herself as she moved into a new stage in life" (he references Gail Sheehy's book *Passages*). He notes that a year ago his wife moved in with an "unemployed alcoholic" although she is currently not living with this man. Mr. Reunter has custody of the children and he states that he is dealing with his own depression related to the loss of his marriage. Mr. Reunter works as a shoe salesman. He wonders if the recent divorce and his own feelings of depression are related to Jason's drop in grades and feelings of depression.

Kenny

Kenny is a 28-year-old male who was referred to this therapist due to feelings of depression as a result of the recent death of a friend from AIDS and the emergence of memories of being molested as a very young child by an adult male relative. In addition, he is currently questioning his sexual identity, which has been homosexual his whole adult life.

Kenny's mood has been depressed. However, despite a suicide attempt by ingestion of pills six months ago, he currently denies suicidal ideation and states he wants to "move on" with his life. Kenny has had a number of recent experiences including seeing flashes of white light, black forms, feelings of something crawling on him, and feeling like he was "shocked." He feels that some of this may be related to feelings of guilt related to a strict fundamentalist upbringing. He states that the guilt he has felt from his homosexual lifestyle may have caused him much stress, which manifested in some of the above symptoms. He describes his homosexual relationships as addictive and compulsive in nature. He has never had a long-term relationship.

Kenny is alert; is oriented to time, place, and person; and is verbal. He is quite open, easily sharing much about his life. He appears to have a moderately depressed mood, and periodically he sobs about the death of his friend, the guilt he feels about his homosexuality, and the memories of his sexual molestation. He seems coherent and his thinking seems clear. His conversations are clear and sharp. Although there is no clear indication of verbal or auditory hallucinations, the fact that he sees white lights and black forms, and feels like things are crawling on him should be explored in more depth as possible hallucinatory material. It is unclear as to whether these are manifestations of a stressful period in his life, are medical in nature, or are possible hallucinations of a psychotic nature. He currently denies suicidal or homicidal ideation.

Appendix G

❖

Generic and Trade Names of Common Medications (Generic/Trade)

Antipsychotic

PHENOTHIAZINES
Chlorpromazine/Thorazine
Triflupromazine/Vesprin
Mesoridazine/Serentil
Piperacetzine/Quide
Thioridazine/Mellaril
Acetophenazine/Tindal
Butaperazine/Repoise
Carphenazine/Proketazine
Fluphenazine/Prolixin
Fluphenazine/Permitil
Perphenazine/Trilafon
Trifluoperazine/Stelazine

THIOXANTHENES
Chlorprohixene/Taractan
Thioxthixene/Navane

BUTYROPHENONES
Haloperidol/Haldol

DIHYDRONIDOLONES
Molindone/Mobane
Molindone/Lidone
Dibenzoxazepines
Loxapine/Loxitane
Loxapine/Daxoline

"ATYPICAL"
Clozapine/Clozaril
Risperidone/Risperdal

Antidepressant

MAOIs
Isocarboxizd/Marplan
Phenelzine/Nardine
Tranylcypromine/Parnate

TRICYCLICS
Amitriptyline/Elavil
Amoxapine/Asendin
Desipramine/Norpramine
Desipramine/Pertofrance
Clomipramine/Anafranil
Imipramine/Tofranil
Maprotiline/Ludiomil
Nortriptyline/Aventyl
Nortriptyline/Pamelor
Protriptyline/Vivactil
Trazodone/Desyrel
Trimipramine/Surmontil

SSRIs
Sertraline/Zoloft
Fluvoxamine/Luvox
Fluvoxamine/Prozac
Paroxetine/Paxil

"ATYPICAL"
Venlafzine/Effexor
Remeron
Nefazodone/Serzone
Bupropion/Wellbutrin

Antianxiety

Alprazolam/Xanax
Chlodiazeoxide/Librax
Chlodiazeoxide/Libritabs
Chlodiazeoxide/Librium
Clorazepate/Azene
Clorazepate/Azene
Clorazepate/Tranxene
Diazepam/Valium
Halazepam/Paxipam
Lorazepam/Ativan
Oxazepam/Serax
Prazepam/Centrax
Buspirone/BuSpar*

Antimanic

Lithium citrate/Cibalith-S
Lithium carbonate/Eskalith
Lithium carbonate/Litane
Lithium carbonate/
Lithobid
Carbamzepine/Tegretol
Carbamzepine/Tegretol
Divalproex sodium/
Depakote

Stimulant

Pemoline/Cylert
Dexedrine/D-amphetamine
Ritalin/Methylphenidate

* BuSpar is the only nonbenzodiazepine. Note: Not all medications are listed. In some cases, rot all trade names are listed.

Appendix H

Example of an Initial Intake Case Report

Demographic Information

Name: Jim Needhelp

Address: Nowhere Land

Phone: 555-5353

Date of Birth: 1/23/75

Date of Interview: 5/21/00

Clinician: Ed Neukrug

Reason for Report

Jim is a 25-year-old single male who was referred to this agency by his mother, who reports that Jim has been hearing things lately and acting "kind of odd." Jim states that he is fine, except that he sometimes hears voices that tell him what's going to happen in the future. He believes he has control over other people's lives through these voices. He states he would like counseling to make him a better person and to get "rid of the voices—maybe."

Background Information

Jim is the youngest of three boys of Jane and Bill. His brother William, Jr., is five years older, married, and has two children. His brother Wally is two years older, single, and living in another state, working in construction. Jim states that he does not work but "does a lot of chores around the house." He reports that his mother, Jane, works part-time at the local convenience store and his dad works at the power plant, doing general "cleanup." He states that his parents have high school educations and that he "almost finished high school but the teachers were mean to me." He states that he wants to get his G.E.D. so that he could obtain a good job. He says that he loves his mother and father, although notes that his father is a "little too strict" at times.

His mother states that Jim has always been a little "odd" and never really had any friends. Jim and his mother state that he was in counseling once before, when he was in high school. His mother reports that it was at this time that she realized Jim heard voices in his head. Jim states that he did have "odd thoughts" at times. He states he always knew that at times he could predict the future and that his thoughts affected the lives of others in unusual ways. When asked specifically if he could give some examples, he refused. Jim stated that he discontinued counseling after he realized his counselor was out to get him, just like everyone else. When asked how, he stated his counselor wanted to put him in the hospital. His mother states that Jim was taking a small dosage of some type of "think right" medication.

Jim states that he thinks it's "weird" that he is 25 years old and still living at home, but notes that he does not think he is capable of living on his own. He spends most of his day watching T.V. and reports that his thoughts can change the ending to the soap operas he watches. When exploring this further, Jim stated that he realizes he is a little odd and is afraid that if he left his home he would get even odder, and "maybe even hurt someone."

Educational and Vocational History

Jim stated that he did not finish high school because he found his teachers "weird." His mother states he was a "slow student" and was tested for a learning disability in reading, but was not coded as disabled. He has a sparse vocational history, noting that he has held jobs for a few months here and there. Most of his jobs have been working part-time at convenience stores or in retail at the local mall. He stated that he usually likes to work, at first, but then the other people where he works begin to "turn on him." He states that he has interest in working, but that for now, he likes being at home, alone.

Medical and Psychiatric History

Jim reports no significant medical history. His mother states that he was six weeks premature and that his doctors were concerned about possible brain damage. However, she reports that he was "perfectly fine." Jim was in counseling for one year with Dr. Shrink and was medicated with what his mother states was a "think right" medication. When asked if this might have been an antipsychotic, she stated that she thought so, but was not sure. His mother stated that Dr. Shrink did discuss with her the possibility of hospitalizing Jim to observe him and monitor his medication. However, she noted that "nobody was going to put my little Jimmy in the hospital."

Mental Status

Jim was dressed in jeans with his shirt hanging out. He looked a little disheveled and there was a strong smell of body odor. He avoided eye contact but was pleasant during the interview. He was oriented to time, place, and person. He responded to questions directly and somewhat concretely. He showed evidence of loose associations and tangential thinking as at times he would ramble about unrelated topics and jump from topic to topic. He denies having visual hallucinations but notes that at times he hears a voice in his head telling him what's going to happen in the future, and he believes he has control over other people's lives through these voices. His affect seemed inappropriate at times, as evidenced by his sudden laughter during the interview. He denies suicidal and homicidal ideation, but states that if people don't leave him alone, "I will get them." He would not clarify what this means.

Diagnostic Impressions

Axis I: None (Rule Out Schizophrenia, Paranoid Type: 205.30)

Axis II: Schizotypal Personality Disorder (301.22)

Axis III: None

Axis IV: Unemployment, Didn't Finish High School

Axis V: GAF = 25 (highest level over past year)

Summary and Recommendations

This 25-year-old single male was referred by his mother who reports that her son has been hearing things lately and acting "kind of odd." Jim states that he periodically hears voices and that he knows he can predict the future and control other people's lives through these voices.

Jim is the youngest of three boys. He reports that he gets along well with his parents, although his father is "a little strict at times." He has worked sporadically since high school, and appears to have difficulty keeping a job. He has personal hygiene problems; apparently he does not bathe regularly. He is oriented by three, but there is evidence of loose associations, suspiciousness, and possible paranoia. His affect during the session was inappropriate, as he would laugh at odd times. He denies being suicidal but states that if people don't leave him alone, "I will get them." He was in counseling for one year during high school and may have been prescribed antipsychotic medication at that time.

The following is recommended:

1. Possible testing for further psychiatric assessment

2. Review for possible medication

3. Further exploration of family dynamics

4. Individual counseling, 1 time weekly

5. Possible day treatment

6. Explore possible assessment for learning disability

7. Explore possibility of attainment of G.E.D.

Ed Neukrug, Ed.D., LPC.

References

Adler, A. (1964). Social interest: A challenge to mankind. New York: Capricorn.

American Counseling Association (ACA). (1995). *Code of ethics and standards of practice* (rev. ed.). Alexandria, VA: Author.

American Mental Health Counselors Association. (1987). *Code of ethics for mental health counselors.* Alexandria, VA: Author.

American Psychiatric Association. (2000). *Diagnostic and statistical manual of mental disorders,* text revision (4th ed.). Washington, DC: Author.

American Psychological Association (APA). (1992). *Ethical principles of psychologists and code of conduct* (rev. ed.). Washington, DC: Author.

Andelsman, M. M., Kemper, M. B., Kesson-Craig, P., McLain, J., & Johnsrud, C. (1986). Use, content, and readability of written informed consent forms for treatment. *Professional Psychology: Research & Practice, 17*(6), 514–518.

Ansell, C. (1984). Ethical practices workbook. In *Preparatory course for the national and state licensing examinations in psychology* (Vol. IV). Los Angeles: Association for Advanced Training in the Behavioral Sciences.

Appigranesi, R. (1990). Freud for beginners. New York: David McKay Company.

Argyle, M. (1975). *Bodily communication.* London: Methuen.

Association of Counselor Education and Supervision (ACES). (1995). Ethical guidelines for counseling supervisors. *Counselor Education and Supervision, 34,* 270–276.

Atkinson, D. R. (1985). A meta-review of research on cross-cultural counseling and psychotherapy. *Journal of Multicultural Counseling and Development, 13,* 138–153.

Atkinson, D. R., Morten, G., & Sue, D. W. (1993). *Counseling American minorities: A cross-cultural perspective* (4th ed.). Madison, WI: Brown & Benchmark.

Atkinson, D. R., Poston, W. C., Furlong, M. J., & Mercado, P. (1989). Ethnic group preferences for counselor characteristics. *Journal of Counseling Psychology, 36,* 68–72.

Axelson, L. J., & Dail, P. W. (1988). The changing character of homelessness in the United States. *Family Relations, 37,* 463–469.

Baker, S. (1995). Becoming multiculturally competent counselors. *The School Counselor, 42,*179.

Ballenger, J. C. (1996). Benzodiazepines. In A. F. Schatzberg & C. B. Nemeroff (Eds.), *Textbook of psychopharmacology* (pp. 215–230). Washington, DC: American Psychiatric Press.

Benjamin, A. (1987). *The helping interview with case illustrations* (4th ed.). Boston: Houghton Mifflin.

Binswanger, L. (1962). *Existential analysis and psychotherapy.* New York: Dutton.

Binswanger, L. (1963). *Being-in-the-world. Selected papers.* New York: Basic Books.

Blasi, G. L. (1990). Social policy and social science research on homelessness. *Journal of Social Issues, 46*(4), 207–219.

Borders, L. D. (1994). *The good supervisor* (Report No. EDO-CG-94-18). Greensboro, NC: ERIC Clearinghouse on Counseling and Student Services. (ERIC Document Reproduction Service No. ED 372 350)

Bordin, E. S. (1968). *Psychological counseling* (2nd ed.). New York: Appleton-Century-Crofts.

Bordin, E. S. (1979). The generalizability of the psychoanalytic concept of the working alliance. *Psychotherapy: Theory, Research, and Practice, 16,* 252–260.

Bradley, L. J., & Gould, L. J. (1994). Supervisee resistance (Report No. EDO-CG-94-12). Greensboro, NC: ERIC Clearinghouse on Counseling and Student Services. (ERIC Document Reproduction Service No. ED 372-344)

Brammer, L. M., & MacDonald, G. (1998). *The helping relationship* (7th ed.). Boston: Allyn & Bacon.

Bray, J. H., Shepherd, J. N., & Hays, J. R. (1985). Legal and ethical issues in informed consent to psychotherapy. *American Journal of Family Therapy, 13*(2), 50–60.

Brill, A. (1985). *Basic principles of psychoanalysis.* Lanham, MD: University Press of America. (Original work published 1948)

Browning, C., Reynolds, A. L., & Dworkin, S. H. (1995). Affirmative psychotherapy for lesbian women. In D. R. Atkinson, & G. Hackett (Eds.). *Counseling diverse populations* (pp. 289–306). Madison, WI: Brown & Benchmark

Budman, S. H., & Gurman, A. S. (1988). *Theory and practice of brief therapy.* New York: Guilford.

Buscaglia, L. (1972). *Love.* Thorofare, NJ: Slack.

Byrne, R. H. (1995). *Becoming a master counselor: Introduction to the profession.* Pacific Grove, CA: Brooks/Cole.

Carkhuff, R. R. (1969). *Helping and human relations* (Vol. 2). New York: Holt, Rinehart & Winston.

Carkhuff, R. R. (2000). *The art of helping* (8th ed.). Amherst, MA: Human Resource Development Press.

Carkhuff, R. R., & Berenson, B. G. (1977). *Beyond counseling and therapy* (2nd ed.). New York: Holt Rinehart & Winston.

Carson, S. (2000). *The mental status exam.* Retrieved June 7, 2001, from the World Wide Web: http://www.pharmacy.unc.edu/xpharmd/phpr177/carson/mse1.htm

Cass, V. C. (1979). Homosexual identity formation: A theoretical model. *Journal of Homosexuality, 4,* 219–235.

Cayleff, S. E. (1986). Ethical issues in counseling, gender, race, and culturally distinct groups. *Journal of Counseling and Development, 64,* 345–347.

Code of Virginia. (1950). *Communications between physicians and patients,* 8.01–399, p. 439.

Cogan, D. B., & O'Connell, G. R. (1982). Models of supervision: A five-year review of the literature. *Journal of the National Organization of Human Service Educators, 4,* 12–17.

Cole, J., & Pilisuk, M. (1976). Differences in the provision of mental health services by race. *American Journal of Orthopsychiatry, 46,* 520–525.

Committee on Government Operations. (1991). *A citizen's guide on using the Freedom of Information Act and the Privacy Act of 1974 to request government records* (fourth report). (House Report 102–146). Washington, DC: U.S. Government Printing Office.

Conte, H., Plutchik, R., Wild, K., & Karasu, T. (1986). Combined psychotherapy and pharmacotherapy for depressions. *Archives of General Psychiatry, 38,* 471–479.

Copeland, E. J. (1983). Cross-cultural counseling and psychotherapy: A historical perspective, implications for research and training. *Personnel and Guidance Journal, 62,* 10–15.

Cormier, W. H., & Cormier, L. S. (1997). *Interviewing strategies for helpers* (4th ed.). Pacific Grove, CA: Brooks/Cole.

Corey, G. (2001). *Theory and practice of counseling and psychotherapy* (6th ed.). Pacific Grove, CA: Brooks/Cole.

Corey, G., Corey, M., & Callanan, P. (1998). *Issues and ethics in the helping professions* (5th ed.). Pacific Grove, CA: Brooks/Cole.

Cottone, R. R., & Tarvydas, V. M. (1998). *Ethical and professional issues in counseling.* Upper Saddle River, NJ: Merrill.

D'Andrea, M. (1996, November 19). *Multicultural counseling.* Presentation at Old Dominion University, Norfolk, VA.

D'Andrea, M., & Daniels, J. (1991). Exploring the different levels of multicultural counseling training in counselor education. *Journal of Counseling and Development, 70,* 78–85.

Derlega, V. J., Lovell, R., & Chaikin, A. L. (1976). Effects of therapist disclosure and its perceived appropriateness on client self-disclosure. *Journal of Consulting and Clinical Psychology, 44,* 866.

Deutsch, C. J. (1984). Self-reported sources of stress among psychotherapists. *Professional Psychology: Research & Practice, 15,* 833–845.

Donley, R. J., Horan, J. J., & DeShong, R. L. (1990). The effect of several self-disclosure permutations on counseling process and outcome. *Journal of Counseling and Development, 67,* 408–412.

Donlon, P. T., Schaffer, C. B., Ericson, S. E., Rockwell, F. P. A., & Schaffer, L. C. (1983). *A manual of psychotropic drugs: A mental health resource.* Bowie, MD: Robert J. Brady.

Doster, J. A., & Nesbitt, J. G. (1979). Psychotherapy and self-disclosure. In J. Chelune & Associates (Eds.), *Self-disclosure: Origins, patterns, and implications of openness in interpersonal relationships* (pp. 177–242). San Francisco: Jossey-Bass.

Downing, N. E., & Roush, K. L. (1985). From passive acceptance to active commitment: A model of feminist identity development for women. *Counseling Psychologist, 13,* 695–709.

Doyle, R. E. (1997). *Essential skills and strategies in the helping process.* Pacific Grove, CA: Brooks/Cole.

Drum, D. J. (1992). A review of Leo Goldman's article "Qualitative assessment: An approach for counselors." *Journal of Counseling & Development, 70,* 622–623.

Drummond, R. J. (2000). Appraisal procedures for counselors and helping professionals (4th ed.). Columbus, OH: Merrill.

Dryden, W., & Feltham, C. (1992). *Brief counselling: A practical guide for beginning practitioners.* Philadelphia: Open University Press.

Dyne, W. A. (Ed.). (1990). *Encyclopedia of homosexuality: Volume 1.* New York: Garland.

Egan, G. (2001). *The skilled helper* (7th ed.). Pacific Grove, CA: Brooks/Cole.

Erikson, E. H. (1998). The life cycle completed. New York: W. W. Norton.

Essandoh, P. K. (1996). Multicultural counseling as the "fourth force": A call to arms. *Counseling Psychologist, 24,* 126–138.

Evans, D. R., Hearn, M. T., Uhlemann, M. R., & Ivey, A. E. (1993). *Essential interviewing* (4th ed.). Pacific Grove, CA: Brooks/Cole.

Evans, G. W., & Howard, R. B. (1973). Personal space. *Psychological Bulletin, 80, 334–344.*

Fawcett, J., & Busch, K. A. (1996). Stimulants in psychiatry. In A. F. Schatzberg & C. B. Nemeroff (Eds.), *Textbook of psychopharmacology* (pp. 417–438). Washington, DC: American Psychiatric Press.

Fitzgerald, L. F., & Nutt, R. (1995). The division 17 principles concerning the counseling/psychotherapy of women: Rationale and implementation. In D. R. Atkinson & G. Hackett (Eds.), *Counseling diverse populations* (pp. 229–261). Madison, WI: Brown & Benchmark.

Fong, M. L. (1995). Assessment and DSM-IV diagnosis of personality disorders: A primer for counselors. *Journal of Counseling Development, 73,* 635–639.

Foster, S. (1996, January). The consequences of violating the "forbidden zone." *Counseling Today,* p. 24.

Fowler, J. (1981). *Stages of faith: The psychology of human development and the quest for meaning.* New York: Harper & Row.

Freud, S. (1947), The ego and the id. London: Hogarth Press.

Fukuyama, M. A. (1994). Multicultural training: If not now, when? If not you, who? *Counseling Psychologist, 22,* 296–299.

Gabbard, G. O. (1995). What are boundaries in psychotherapy? *The Menninger Letter, 3*(4), 1–2.

Garfield, S. L. (1989). *The practice of brief psychotherapy.* New York: Pergamon Press.

Garretson, D. J. (1993). Psychological misdiagnosis of African Americans. *Journal of Multicultural Counseling and Development, 21,* 119–126.

Gazda, G. M., Asbury, F. R., Balzer, F. J., Childers, W. C., & Phelps, W. C. (1999). *Human relations development: A manual for educators* (6th ed.). Boston: Allyn & Bacon.

Gelso, C. J., & Carter, J. A. (1994). Components of the psychotherapy relationship: Their interaction and unfolding during treatment. *Journal of Counseling Psychology, 41,* 296–306.

George, R. L., & Cristiani, R. S. (1994). *Counseling theory and practice* (4th ed.). Boston: Allyn & Bacon.

Germain, C. B. (1981). The physical environment and social work practice. In A. N. Maluccio (Ed.), *Promoting competence in clients* (pp. 103–124). New York: Free Press.

Gibson, R. L., & Mitchell, M. H. (1995). *Introduction to counseling and guidance* (4th ed.). Englewood Cliffs, NJ: Merrill.

Gladding, S. (1996). *Community and agency counseling.* Upper Saddle River, NJ: Prentice-Hall.

Gladstein, G. (1983). Understanding empathy: Integrating counseling, developmental, and social psychology perspectives. *Journal of Counseling Psychology, 30,* 467–482.

Goldman, L. (1992). Qualitative assessment: An approach for counselors. *Journal of Counseling & Development, 70,* 616–621.

Goldstein, A. P. (1980). Relationship-enhancement methods. In F. H. Kanfer & A. P. Goldstein (Eds.), *Helping people change* (pp. 18–57). New York: Pergamon Press.

Gompertz, K. (1960). The relation of empathy to effective communication. *Journalism Quarterly, 37,* 535–546.

Greenberg, L. S. (1994). What is "real" in the relationship? Comment on Gelso and Carter (1994). *Journal of Counseling Psychology, 41,* 307–309.

Greenberg, R. P., & Staller, J. (1981). Personal therapy for therapists. *American Journal of Psychiatry, 138,* 1461–1471.

Gutheil, I. A. (1991). The physical environment and quality of life in residential facilities for frail elders. *Adult Residential Care Journal, 5,* 131–145.

Hackney, H. L., & Cormier, L. S. (2000). *The professional counselor: A process guide to helping* (4th ed.). Needham Heights, MA: Allyn & Bacon.

Handelsman, M. M., Kemper, M. B., Kesson-Craig, P., McLain, J., & Johnsrud, C. (1986). Use, content, and readability of written informed consent forms for treatment. *Professional Psychology: Research & Practice, 17,* 514–518.

Hansen, J. C., Stevie, R. R., & Warner, R. W. (1987). Counseling: Theory and process. Boston: Allyn & Bacon.

Harrington, T. F. (1995). *Assessment of abilities.* (Report No. EDO-CG-95-12). Greensboro, NC: ERIC Clearinghouse on Counseling and Student Services. (ERIC Document Reproduction Service No. ED 389 960)

Hashimi, J. (1991). Counseling older adults. In P. K. H. Kim (Ed.), *Serving the elderly: Skills for practice* (pp. 33–51). New York: McGraw-Hill.

Herlihy, B., & Corey, G. (1997). *Boundary issues in counseling: Multiple roles and responsibilities.* Alexandria, VA: American Counseling Association.

Hersen, M., & Van Hasselt, V. B. (Eds.). (1994). *Advanced abnormal psychology.* New York: Plenum Press.

Highlen, P. S., & Hill, C. E. (1984). Factors affecting client change in individual counseling. In S. D. Brown & R. W. Lent (Eds.), *Handbook of counseling psychology* (pp. 334–396). New York: Wiley.

Hinkle, S. (1994a). *Psychodiagnosis for counselors: The DSM-IV.* (Report No. MF01/PC01). Greensboro, NC: ERIC Clearinghouse on Counseling and Student Services. (ERIC Document Reproduction Service No. ED 366 890)

Hinkle, S. (1994b). The DSM-IV: Prognosis and implications for mental health counselors. *Journal of Mental Health Counseling, 16*(2), 174–183.

Hohenshil, T. H. (1993). Assessment and diagnosis in the Journal of Counseling and Development. *Journal of Counseling and Development, 72,* 7.

Hohenshil. T. H. (1994). DSM-IV: What's new. *Journal of Counseling & Development, 73,* 105–107.

Horst, E. A. (1995). Reexamining gender issues in Erikson's stages of identity and intimacy. *Journal of Counseling and Development, 73,* 271–278.

Hutchins, D. E., & Cole, C. G. (1992). *Helping relationships and strategies* (2nd ed.). Pacific Grove, CA: Brooks/Cole.

Ivey, A., & Ivey, M. (1998). *Intentional interviewing and counseling* (4rd ed.). Pacific Grove, CA: Brooks/Cole.

Jaffee v. Redmond, (95-266), 518 U.S. 1 (1996).

Jayakar, P. (1986). *Krishnamurti: A biography.* New York: Harper & Row.

Jourard, S. M. (1971). *The transparent self: Self disclosure and well-being* (2nd ed.). Princeton, NJ: Van Nostrand Reinhold.

Jung, C. G. (1968). *Analytical psychology: Its theory and practice: The Tavistock lectures.* New York: Pantheon Books (Original Work Published in 1935).

Jung, C. G. (1975). Freud and Jung: Contrasts. In R. F. C. Hull (Trans.). *Critiques of Psychoanalysis.* (Extracted from *The Collected Works of C. G. Jung* (Vols. 4 and 18) by W. McGuire, Ed., 1961, Princeton, NJ: Princeton University Press. (Original Work Published in 1929)

Kahn, M. (1991). *Between therapist and client: The new relationship.* New York: W. H. Freeman.

Kanfer, F. H., & Goldstein, A. P. (Eds.). (1991). *Helping people change* (4th ed.). Needham Heights, MA: Allyn & Bacon.

Kazantzakis, N. (1952). *Zorba the Greek.* New York: Simon & Schuster.

Kelly, K. R., & Hall, A. S. (Eds.). (1992). Mental health counseling for men. [Special issue]. *Journal of Mental Health Counseling, 19*(2).

Kitchener, K. S. (1984). Intuition, critical evaluation and ethical principles: The foundation for ethical decisions in counseling psychology. *Counseling Psychologist, 12,* 43–45.

Kleinke, C. L. (1994). *Common principles of psychotherapy.* Pacific Grove, CA: Brooks/Cole.

Kohut, H. (1984). How does analysis cure? Chicago: University of Chicago Press.

Kramer, P. D. (1997). *Listening to Prozac.* New York: Penguin Books.

Kübler-Ross, E. (1997). *On death and dying.* New York: Simon & Schuster.

Lambert, M. J., & Bergin, A. E. (1983). Therapist characteristics and their contribution to psychotherapy outcome. In C. E. Walker (Ed.), *Handbook of psychotherapy and behavior change* (pp. 205–241). Homewood, IL: Dow Jones-Irwin.

Lambert, M. J., Shapiro, D. A., & Bergin, A. E. (1986). The effectiveness of psychotherapy. In S. L. Garfield & A. E. Bergin (Eds.), *Handbook of psychotherapy and behavior change* (pp. 157–211). New York: Wiley.

Lee, C. C. (1994). Pioneers of multicultural counseling: A conversation with Clemmont E. Vontress. *Journal of Multicultural Counseling and Development, 22,* 66–78.

Lee, W. M. L., & Mixson, R. J. (1995). Asian and Caucasian client perceptions of the effectiveness of counseling. *Journal of Multicultural Counseling and Development, 23,* 48–56.

Levinson, D. (1986). *The seasons of a man's life.* New York: Ballantine.

Linzer, N. (1990). Ethics and human service practice. *Human Service Education, 10*(1), 15–22.

Locke, D. (1992). Counseling beyond U.S. borders. *American Counselor, 1,* 13–17.

Loewenberg, F., & Dolgoff, R. (1996). *Ethical decisions for social work practice* (5th ed.). Itasca, IL: Peacock.

Lombana, J. H. (1989). Counseling persons with disabilities: Summary and projections. *Journal of Counseling and Development, 68,* 177–179.

Loulan, J. (1987). *Lesbian passion: Loving ourselves and each other.* San Francisco: Spinsters/Aunt Lute.

Lynn S. J., & Garske, P. J. (Eds.). (1990). *Contemporary psychotherapies: Models and methods.* Upper Saddle River, NJ: Prentice-Hall.

Mabe, A. R., & Rollin, S. A. (1986). The role of a code of ethical standards in counseling. *Journal of Counseling and Development, 64,* 294–297.

Marder, S. R., & Van Putten, T. (1996). Antipsychotic medications. In A. F. Schatzberg & C. B. Nemeroff (Eds.), *Textbook of psychopharmacology* (pp. 247–262). Washington, DC: American Psychiatric Press.

Maslow, A. (1970). *Motivation and personality* (rev. ed.) New York: Harper & Row.

Maslow, A. (1998). *Toward a psychology of being* (3rd ed.). New York: Wiley.

McElroy, S. L., & Keck, P. E. (1996). Antiepileptic drugs. In A. F. Schatzberg & C. B. Nemeroff (Eds.), Textbook of psychopharmacology (pp. 351–376). Washington, DC: American Psychiatric Press, Inc.

McGoldrick, M., Pearce, J. K., & Giordano, J. (1996). *Ethnicity and family therapy* (2nd ed.). New York: Guilford Press.

McNamara, K., & Rickard, K. M. (1989). Feminist identity development: Implications for feminist therapy with women. *Journal of Counseling and Development, 68,* 184–189.

Mehrabian, A. (1972). *Nonverbal communication.* Chicago: Aldene-Atherton.

Midgette, T. E., & Meggert, S. S. (1991). Multicultural counseling instruction: A challenge for faculties in the 21st century. *Journal of Counseling and Development, 70,* 136–141.

Minuchin, S. (1974). *Families and family therapy.* Cambridge, MA: Harvard University Press.

Moore, D., & Haverkamp, B. E. (1989). Measured increases in male emotional expressiveness following a structured group intervention. *Journal of Counseling and Development, 67,* 513–517.

Morse, P. S., & Ivey, A. E. (1996). *Face to face: Communication and conflict resolution in the schools.* Thousand Oaks, CA: Corwin Press.

Mwaba, K., & Pedersen, P. (1990). Relative importance of intercultural, interpersonal, and psychopathological attributions in judging critical incidents by multicultural counselors. *Journal of Multicultural Counseling and Development, 18,* 106–117.

National Association of Social Workers (NASW). (1996). *Revised code of ethics of the National Association of Social Workers.* Washington, DC: Author.

National Institute of Mental Health. (1995). *Decade of the brain* (3rd ed.). [Brochure]. Rockville, MD: Author.

National Opinion Research Center. (1991). *General social surveys, 1972–1991: Cumulative codebook.* Chicago: Author.

National Organization of Human Service Education. (1995). Ethical standards of human service professionals. Retrieved May 1, 2001, from the World Wide Web: http://nohse.com/ethstand.html.

Neimeyer, G. J., Banikiotes, P. G., & Winum, P. C. (1979). Self-disclosure flexibility and counseling-related perceptions. *Journal of Counseling Psychology, 26,* 546–548.

Neimeyer, G. J., & Fong, M. L. (1983). Self-disclosure flexibility and counselor effectiveness. *Journal of Counseling Psychology, 30,* 258–261.

Neukrug, E. (1980). *The effects of supervisory style and type of praise upon counselor trainees' level of empathy and perception of supervisor.* Unpublished doctoral dissertation, University of Cincinnati, Cincinnati, OH.

Neukrug, E. (1987). The brief training of paraprofessional counselors in empathic responding. *New Hampshire Journal for Counseling and Development, 15*(1), 15–19.

Neukrug, E. (1994). Understanding diversity in a pluralistic world. *The Journal of Intergroup Relations, 21(2),* 3–12.

Neukrug, E. (1996). A developmental approach to the teaching of ethical decision making. *Human Service Education, 16*(1), pp. 19–36.

Neukrug, E. (1997). Support and challenge: Use of metaphor as a higher level empathic response. In H. Rosenthal (Ed.), *Favorite counseling and therapy techniques* (pp. 139–141). Bristoll, PA: Accelerated Development.

Neukrug, E. (1999a). *The world of the counselor.* Pacific Grove, CA: Brooks/Cole.

Neukrug, E. (1999b). *The world of the counselor: An experiential workbook for developing professional competencies.* Pacific Grove, CA: Brooks/Cole.

Neukrug, E. (2000). *Theory, practice and trends in human services: An introduction to an emerging profession* (2nd ed.). Pacific Grove, CA: Brooks/Cole.

Neukrug, E., & McAuliffe, G. (1993). Cognitive development and human service education. *Human Service Education, 13*(1), 13–26.

Neukrug, E., & Williams, G. (1993). Counseling counselors: A survey of values. *Counseling and Values, 38*(1), 51–62.

Neukrug, E., Lovell, C., & Parker, R. (1996). Employing ethical codes and decision-making models: A developmental process. *Counseling and Values, 40,* 98–106.

Neukrug, E., Milliken, T., & Shoemaker, J. (2001). Counselor seeking behaviors of NOHSE practitioners, educators, and trainees. *Human Service Education,* 21. In Press.

Neukrug, E., Milliken, T., & Walden, S. (2001). Ethical complaints made against licensed professional counselors. Counselor Education and Supervision. In Press.

Nishino, S., Mignot, E., & Dement, W. C. (1996). Sedative-hypnotics. In A. F. Schatzberg & C. B. Nemeroff (Eds.), *Textbook of psychopharmacology* (pp. 405–416). Washington, DC: American Psychiatric Press.

Norcross, J. C., Strausser, D. J., & Faltus, F. J. (1988). The therapist's therapist. *American Journal of Psychotherapy, 42*(1), 53–66.

Norden, M. J. (1996). *Beyond Prozac: Brain-toxic lifestyles, natural antidotes and new generation antidepressants* (2nd ed.). New York: ReganBooks.

Nurius, P. S., & Hudson, W. (1989a). Computers and social diagnosis: The client's perspective. *Computers in the Human Services, 5*(1–2), 21–35.

Nurius, P. S., & Hudson, W. (1989b). Workers, clients, and computers. *Computers in Human Services, 4*(1–2), 71–83.

Orlinsky, D. E., & Howard, K. I. (1986). Process and outcome in psychotherapy. In S. L. Garfield & A. E. Bergin (Eds.), *Handbook of psychotherapy and behavior change* (3rd ed., pp. 311–381). New York: Wiley.

Osherson, S. (1986). *Finding our fathers.* New York: Faucett Columbine.

Peck, M. S. (1998). *People of the lie.* New York: Simon & Schuster.

Pedersen, P. (2000). *A handbook for developing multicultural awareness* (3rd ed.). Alexandria, VA: American Counseling Association.

Pedersen, P. B., Draguns, J. G., Lonner, W. J., & Trimble, J. E. (1996). *Counseling across cultures* (4th ed.). Thousand Oaks, CA: Sage.

Pennebaker, J. W., Colder, M., & Sharp, L. K. (1990). Accelerating the coping process. *Journal of Personality and Social Psychology, 58,* 528–537.

Pennebaker, J. W., & Susman, J. R. (1988). Disclosure of traumas and psychosomatic processes. *Social Science and Medicine, 26,* 327–332.

Perry, M. A., & Furukawa, M. J. (1986). Modeling methods. In F. H. Kanfer & A. P. Goldstein (Eds.), *Helping people change: A textbook of methods* (3rd ed., pp. 66–110). New York: Pergamon Press.

Pope, M. (1995). The "salad bowl" is big enough for us all: An argument for the inclusion of lesbians and gay men in any definition of multiculturalism. *Journal of Counseling and Development, 73,* 301–303.

Pope, K. S., & Tabachnick, B. G. (1993). Therapists' anger, hate, fear, and sexual feelings: National survey of therapist response characteristics, client characteristics, critical events, formal complaints, and training. *Professional Psychology: Research and Practice, 24,* 142–152.

Pope, K. S., & Tabachnik, B. G. (1994). Therapists as patients: A national survey of psychologists' experiences, problems, and beliefs. *Professional Psychology Research and Practice, 25*(3), 247–258.

Poston, W. S. C., Craine, M., & Atkinson, D. R. (1991). Counselor dissimilarity, confrontation, client cultural mistrust, and willingness to self-disclose. *Journal of Multicultural Counseling and Development, 19,* 65–73.

Preston, J., Varzos, N., & Liebert, D. S. (2000). *Every session counts: Making the most out of your brief therapy* (2nd ed.). Oakland, CA: New Harbinger Publications.

Prochaska, J. O., & Norcross, J. C. (1983). Contemporary psychotherapists: A national survey of characteristics, practices, orientations, and attitudes. *Psychotherapy: Theory, Research and Practice, 20*(2), 161–173.

Proshansky, H. M., Ittleson, W. H., & Rivlin, L. G. (1970). The influence of the physical environment on behavior: Some basic assumptions. In H. M. Proshansky, W. H. Ittleson, & L. G. Rivlin (Eds.), *Environmental psychology: Man and his physical setting* (pp. 27–37). New York: Holt, Rinehart & Winston.

Quintana, S. M., & Bernal, M. E. (1995). Ethnic minority training in counseling psychology: Comparison with clinical psychology and proposed standards. *The Counseling Psychologist, 23*(1), 102–121.

Raskind, M. A. (1996). Treatment of Alzheimer's disease and other dementias. In A. F. Schatzberg & C. B. Nemeroff (Eds.), *Textbook of psychopharmacology* (pp. 657–668). Washington, DC: American Psychiatric Press, Inc.

Remley, R. P., Herlihy, B., & Herlihy, S. B. (1997). The U. S. Supreme Court decision in *Jaffe v. Redmond:* Implications for counselors. *Journal of Counseling and Development, 75,* 213–218.

Reynolds, J. F., Mair, D. C., & Fischer, P. C. (1995). *Writing and reading mental health records: Issues and analysis* (2nd ed.). Mahwah, NJ: Erlbaum Associates.

Rogers, C. R. (1942). *Counseling and psychotherapy: New concepts in practice.* Boston: Houghton Mifflin.

Rogers, C. R. (1957). The necessary and sufficient conditions of therapeutic personality change. *Journal of Counseling Psychology, 21*(2), 95–103.

Rogers, C. R. (1959). A theory of therapy, personality and interpersonal relationships as developed in the client-centered framework. In S. Koch (Ed.), *Psychology: A study of science: Vol. 3. Formulations of the person and the social context* (pp. 184–256). New York: McGraw-Hill.

Rogers, C. R. (1961). Ellen West—and loneliness. In H. Kirschenbaum & V. L. Henderson (Eds.), *The Carl Rogers reader* (pp. 157–167). Boston: Houghton Mifflin.

Rogers, C. R. (1970). *Carl Rogers on encounter groups.* New York: Harper & Row.

Rogers, C. R. (1980). *A way of being.* Boston: Houghton Mifflin.

Rogers, C. R. (1989). A Client-centered/person-centered approach to therapy. In H. Kirschenbaum (Ed.), *The Carl Rogers reader* (pp. 135–152). Boston: Houghton Mifflin. (Original work published in 1986)

Romano, G. (1992). Description of D. Locke's "Counseling beyond U.S. borders." *American Counselor, 1*(2), 13–17.

Rossi, P. H. (1990). The old homeless and the new homelessness in historical perspective. *American Psychologist, 45*(8), 954–959.

Rowe, W., Murphy, H. B., & De Csipkes, R. A. (1975). The relationship of counseling characteristics and counseling effectiveness. *Review of Educational Research, 45,* 231–246.

Sadow, D., Ryder, M., Stein, J., & Geller, M. (1987). Supervision of mental health students in the context of an educational milieu. *Human Service Education, 8*(2), 29–36.

Safran, J. D., & Segal, Z. V. (1996). *Interpersonal processes in cognitive therapy.* Northvale, NJ: Jason Aronson.

Sandhu, D. S. (1995). Pioneers of multicultural counseling: A conversation with Paul B. Pedersen. *Journal of Multicultural Counseling and Development, 23,* 198–211.

Schatzberg, A. F., & Nemeroff, C. B. (1998). *Textbook of psychopharmacology* (2nd ed.). Washington, DC: American Psychiatric Press.

Scher, M. (1979). On counseling men. *Personnel and Guidance Journal, 57,* 252–254.

Scher, M. (1981). Men in hiding. *Personnel and Guidance Journal, 60,* 199–202.

Schlossberg, N. K. (1995). *Counseling adults in transition* (2nd ed.). New York: Springer.

Schmolling, P., Youkeles, M., & Burger, W. R. (1993). *Human services in contemporary America* (3rd ed.). Pacific Grove, CA: Brooks/Cole.

Schram, B., & Mandel, B. R. (1996). An introduction to human services: Policy and practice (3rd ed.). Needham Heights, MA: Allyn & Bacon.

Scissons, E. D. (1993). *Counseling for results.* Pacific Grove, CA: Brooks/Cole.

Sexton, T. (1993). A review of the counseling outcome research. In G. R. Walz & J. C. Bleuer (Eds.), *Counselor efficacy: Assessing and using counseling outcomes research* (Report No. ISBN-1-56109-056-5). Ann Arbor, MI: ERIC Clearinghouse on Counseling and Personnel Services. (ERIC Document Reproduction Service No. ED 362 821)

Sexton, T., & Whiston, S. C. (1991). A review of the empirical basis for counseling: Implications for practice and training. *Counselor Education and Supervision, 30,* 330–354.

Sexton, T., & Whiston, S. C. (1994). The status of the counseling relationship: An empirical review, theoretical implications, and research directions. *The Counseling Psychologist, 22,* 6–78.

Shannon, J. W., & Woods, W. J. (1995). Affirmative psychotherapy for gay men. In D. R. Atkinson & G. Hackett (Eds.), *Counseling diverse populations* (pp. 307–324). Madison, WI: Brown & Benchmark.

Shipp, P. (1983). Counseling blacks: A group approach. *The Personnel and Guidance Journal,* 108–111.

Shostrum, E. (1974). *Manual for the Personal Orientation Inventory: An inventory for the measurement of self-actualization.* San Diego: Educational and Industrial Testing Service.

Sodowsky, G. R., & Taffe, R. C. (1991). Counselor trainees' analysis of multicultural counseling videotapes. *Journal of Multicultural Counseling and Development, 19,* 115–129.

Solomon, A. (1992). Clinical diagnosis among diverse populations: A multicultural perspective. *Families in Society: The Journal of Contemporary Human Services, 73*(6), 371–377.

Somer, E., & Saadon, M. (1999). Therapist-client sex: Clients' retrospective reports. *Professional Psychology—Research and Practice, 30*(5), 504–509.

Sommer, R. (1959). Studies in personal space. *Sociometry, 22,* 247–260.

Speight, S. L., Myers, J., Cox, C. I., & Highlen, P. S. (1991). A redefinition of multicultural counseling. *Journal of Counseling and Development, 70,* 29–36.

Spiegler, M. D. & Guevremont, D. C. (1998). Contemporary behavior therapy (3rd ed.). Pacific Grove, CA: Brook/Cole.

Steinem, G. (1992). *Revolution from within: A book on self-esteem.* Boston: Little, Brown.

SREB (Southern Regional Educational Board). (1969). Roles and functions of different levels of mental health workers. Atlanta, GA: Author.

Steward, R. J., Neil, D., Jo, H., Hill, M., & Baden, A. (1998). White counselor trainees: Is there multicultural counseling competence without formal training? (Report No.CG028424). Ann Arbor, MI: ERIC Clearinghouse on Counseling and Personnel Services. (ERIC Document Reproduction Service No. ED 419 188)

Sue, D. (1978). Counseling across cultures. *Personnel and Guidance Journal, 56,* 451.

Sue, D. W., & Sue, D. (1990). *Counseling the culturally different: Theory and practice* (2nd ed.). New York: Wiley.

Sue, D. W., Arredondo, P., & McDavis, R. J. (1992). Multicultural counseling competencies and standards: A call to the profession. *Journal of Counseling and Development, 70,* 477–486.

Sue, D. W., Bernier, J. E., Durran, A., Feinberg, L., Pedersen, P., Smith, E. J., & Vasquez-Nuttall, E. (1982). Professional forum: Position paper: Cross-cultural counseling competencies. *Counseling Psychologist, 10,* 45–52.

Sullivan, W., Wolk, J., & Harmann, D. (1992). Case management in alcohol and drug treatment: Improving client outcome. *Families in Society: The Journal of Contemporary Human Services, 73,* 195–204.

Swenson, L. C. (1997). *Psychology and law for the helping professions* (2nd ed.). Pacific Grove, CA: Brooks/Cole.

Swenson, L. C. (1997). *Psychology and law for the helping professions* (2nd ed.). Pacific Grove, CA: Brooks/Cole.

Tafoya, T. (1996, June). *New heights in human services: Multiculturalism.* Keynote address at National Organization of Human Services Annual Conference, St. Louis, MO.

Tarasoff v. Regents of University of California, 529 P.2d 553 (Calif. 1974), vacated, reheard en banc, and affirmed 551 P.2d 334 (1976).

Taylor, M., Bradley, V., & Warren, R. (Eds.). (1996). *The community support skill standards: Tools for managing change and achieving outcomes: Skill standards for direct service workers in the human services.* Cambridge, MA: Human Services Research Institute.

Thompson, J. J. (1973). *Beyond words: Nonverbal communication in the classroom.* New York: Citation Press.

Thompson, R. (1996). *Counseling techniques: Improving relationships with others, ourselves, our families and our environment.* Washington, DC: Accelerated Development.

Tiedeman, D. V. (1983). Flexible filing, computers, and growing. *Counseling Psychologist, 11*, 33–47.

Tollefson, G. D. (1996). Selective serotonin reuptake inhibitors. In A. F. Schatzberg & C. B. Nemeroff (Eds.), *Textbook of psychopharmacology* (pp. 161–183). Washington, DC: American Psychiatric Press.

Truax, C. B., & Mitchell, K. M. (1971). Research on certain therapist interpersonal skills in relation to process and outcome. In A. E. Bergin & S. L. Garfield (Eds.), *Handbook of psychotherapy and behavior change: An empirical analysis.* New York: Wiley.

U.S. Department of Commerce, Bureau of Census. (1996). *Percent of the population, by race and Hispanic origin: 1990, 2000, 2025, and 2050.* Retrieved October 1, 2000, from the World Wide Web: http://www.census.gov/ft. . .popprofile/natproj.html

Vacc, N. A. (1982). A conceptual framework for continuous assessment of clients. *Measurement and Evaluation in Guidance, 15*(1), 40–47.

VanZandt, C. E. (1990). Professionalism: A matter of personal initiative. *Journal of Counseling and Development, 68*, 243–245.

Wakefield, J. C. (1992). The concept of mental disorder: On the boundary between biological facts and social values. *American Psychologist, 47*, 373–388.

Watzlawick, P. (1967). *Pragmatics of human communication.* New York: W. W. Norton.

Westwood, M. J., & Ishiyama, F. I. (1990). The communication process as a critical intervention for client change in cross-cultural counseling. *Journal of Multicultural Counseling and Development, 18*, 163–171.

Wheeler, S. (1991). Personal therapy: An essential aspect of counsellor training, or a distraction from focussing on the client. *Journal for the Advancement of Counselling, 14*, 193–202.

Whiston, S. C., & Coker, J. K. (2000). Reconstructing clinical training: Implications from research. *Counselor Education and Supervision, 39*, 228–253.

Whitfield, D. (1994). Toward an integrated approach to improving multicultural counselor education. *Journal of Multicultural Counseling and Development, 22*, 227–238.

Wicks, R. J. (1993). *Counseling strategies and interventions techniques for the human services* (4th ed.). New York: J. B. Lippincott.

Williams, R. C., & Myer, R. A. (1992). The men's movement: An adjunct to traditional counseling approaches. *Journal of Mental Health Counseling, 14*, 393–404.

Wilson, L. L., & Stith, L. L. (1991). Culturally sensitive therapy with black clients. *Journal of Multicultural Counseling and Development, 19*, 32–43. (Original work published in 1991)

Wolfgang, A. (1985). The function and importance of nonverbal behavior in intercultural counseling. In P. B. Pedersen (Ed.), *Handbook of cross-cultural counseling and therapy* (pp. 99–105). Westport, CT: Greenwood Press.

Woodside, M., & McClam, T. (1998). *Generalist case management: A method of human service delivery.* Pacific Grove, CA: Brooks/Cole.

Wylie, M. S. (1995, September/October). The new visionaries. *The Family Therapy Networker*, pp. 20–29, 32–35.

Young, F. A. (1992). APA and (AP)². *Professional Psychology: Research and Practice, 23*, 436–438.

Yutrzenka, B. A. (1995). Making a case for training in ethnic and cultural diversity in increasing treatment efficacy. *Journal of Consulting and Clinical Psychology, 63*(2), 197–296.

Index